THE HEALTH CARE SUPERVISOR'S CASEBOOK

Charles R. McConnell

Vice President for Employee Affairs
The Genesee Hospital
Rochester, N.Y.

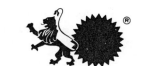

AN ASPEN PUBLICATION®
Aspen Systems Corporation
Rockville, Maryland
London
1982

Library of Congress Cataloging in Publication Data

McConnell, Charles R.
The health care supervisor's casebook.

Includes index.
1. Health facilities—Administration—Case studies.
2. Health services administrators—Case studies.
I. Title. [DNLM: 1. Health facility administrators—
Problems. 2. Hospital administration—Problems.
WX 18 M477h]
RA971.M433 1982   362.1′068′3   82-8875
ISBN: 0-89443-699-6   AACR2

Publisher: John Marozsan
Editorial Director: Michael Brown
Managing Editor: Margot Raphael
Editorial Services: Dorothy Okoroji
Printing and Manufacturing: Debbie Collins

Library of Congress Catalog Card Number: 82-8875
ISBN: 0-89443-699-6

Printed in the United States of America

1 2 3 4 5

Table of Contents

Preface .... **v**

Chapter 1—How To Use the *Casebook* **1**
    Introducing the *Casebook* 1
    Uses of the *Casebook* 1
    One Tool in the Training Kit 3
    The Nature of the Case-Study Approach 5

Chapter 2—The Supervisor's Essential Qualities: All Two of Them **7**
    Only Two? 7
    Courage 8
    Compassion 9
    The Balancing Act 9

Chapter 3—The Emphasis: Determining What's Important to the
    Supervisor **11**
    Background 11
    Forced-Choice Pairs, Applied 15
    Supervisory Topic-Preference Survey 18
    Casebook Topic Emphasis 21

Chapter 4—Introduction to Cases **23**
    Three Views of the Supervisor's Job 23
    Classification of Cases 25
    The *Casebook* Emphasis 26
    Topic Numbering and Cross-Reference 26
    An Example 31
    A Sample Case 31

Chapter 5—Cases in Health Care Supervision **37**

Chapter 6—"The Threat": A Major Case in Interpersonal Relations **137**
    The Setting   137
    The People   137
    The Situation   139
    And Having Done So   144
    "The Threat": Continued   145

Chapter 7—The In-Basket Exercise **149**
    A Comprehensive Exercise   149
    Features   150
    Uses   151
    Developing an In-Basket Exercise   152
    Sample In-Basket Exercise   153

Chapter 8—Introduction to Questions **165**
    Using the Questions   165
    An Example   166

Chapter 9—Questions from Health Care Supervisors **169**

Chapter 10—What Can You Get from All This? **185**
    Practice   185
    New Problem-Solving Outlook   185
    Broadened View   187
    The Benefits of the Case Method   188

Chapter 11—Collecting Your Own Cases **189**
    Sources of Case Material   189
    Fact in Fictional Form   190
    Keep it Simple   191

Index **193**

Preface

I've been a believer in the case-study approach to education since I was first exposed to it in my undergraduate days. Early in my business education, I came to regard the case method as a most useful way to carry classroom fundamentals and textbook principles a few steps closer to the reality of the working world. Perhaps, then, it was only natural that when I began teaching I turned to the case method to supplement other techniques of instruction.

When I began working with health care supervisors, I started looking for cases to use in my classes. I soon found I wasn't simply looking for cases—I was *scratching* for them. A number of cases were available from various sources, but most of these involved the making of investment and marketing decisions in profit-centered industries. Cases applicable to lower and middle managers in health institutions were few and far between. I found I was usually limited to cases that appeared singly in occasional newsletters and journals, or to cases that existed in ones and twos as created by other instructors.

Taking a cue from a few other instructors, I began writing my own cases. Once I became thoroughly involved in the process, I discovered that I would never again have to be overly concerned with the question of where to get case material. I had opened up two major sources: my own experiences and—especially—the questions, problems, and experiences of the supervisors in my classes.

The *Health Care Supervisor's Casebook* consists of cases and questions collected and written during ten years of working with health care supervisors as an instructor and discussion leader. My "students" (if I may call them such since outside of the classroom many have been my friends and coworkers) have given me a wealth of usable case material. They have also taught me that students and their experiences can be an instructor's most valuable source of learning, and that to be effective a teacher must first, foremost, and forever be a student.

Chapter 1

How To Use the *Casebook*

INTRODUCING THE *CASEBOOK*

This is a collection of cases and other aids intended for use in the training and continuing education of health care supervisors. It was developed from the questions and experiences—problems, frustrations, and positive experiences alike—of supervisors actively working in health care organizations.

The *Casebook* stands on its own as a text for supervisory training programs and as a resource for other management development activities. However, it is also intended to supplement more basic texts dealing primarily with principles and fundamentals. Thus you may use the *Casebook* by itself or in conjunction with basic texts such as *The Effective Health Care Supervisor* (Aspen, 1982) or *The Health Care Supervisor's Handbook* (Aspen, 1978).

USES OF THE *CASEBOOK*

Self-study

The *Casebook* can be used for self-study, for example, individual continuing education. Although the role-plays and a limited number of other group-oriented activities are more appropriate to classroom situations, most of the cases and questions may be considered in their entirety by an individual working alone. Simply pick a topic of interest and look up a case or some questions related to that topic.

Assume, for instance, that you face a problem dealing with delegation and that this problem raises some questions concerning the process of delegation. Look up "delegation" directly in the case listings, or begin with the index and trace it through its various references throughout the book.

You need only select a topic of interest, look up pertinent references, and consider the topic at your own pace. You will not immediately find specific answers. However, by considering the questions and cases related to your topic you will broaden your perspective, and the process of doing so may well provide the thought starter you need to solve your problem. Or perhaps the *Casebook* will help you to define your problem more clearly, thus enabling you to decide where you should seek a specific solution.

As compared with the traditional textbook approach, the *Casebook* gives you the "problems at the end of the chapter"—without giving you the chapter. Thus, one approach you might consider is to wrestle with a problem of interest and later analyze your solution. For instance, again assuming your interest in the topic of delegation, you might look up a single delegation case that appears to contain some of the elements in which you are interested. Study the chosen case and develop the best possible solution under the circumstances. Then turn to another resource, perhaps a chapter on the fundamentals of delegation in a basic text on health care supervision, and see how well your solution aligns with theory and principles. If your solution seems to fit, pat yourself on the back. If it seems as though you went astray of the fundamentals, try another case in delegation—and another, and another if necessary—until you can see that the principles of proper delegation are reflected in your solutions.

Alternatively, simply use the *Casebook* as a topic reference. As mentioned earlier, you won't find many specific answers, but you will often find in the questions and problems of others the seeds of the solution to your problem.

Small-Group Activity

A particular hospital department head made it a practice of getting together once each week with the four supervisors who reported to him. They met on the same day each week in a private dining room and considered, informally, a case study which had been assigned the week before. This had been the department head's idea, but participation was optional. Each supervisor took the case of the week, analyzed it, and developed a tentative solution expressed in a paragraph or two. Over lunch the group discussed the five solutions—the department head participated as well—

and developed one solution agreeable to them all. The five managers took turns selecting the case for the following week. More often than not the cases came from problems they encountered in their own departmental units.

The *Casebook* can be used in the same fashion, as material for informal, small-group management development activity. The setting, of course, need not be lunch time in a private dining room. The place could just as well be a conference room or some manager's office, and the time could be a portion of the time allotted to a staff meeting.

Many managers make it a practice to reserve a portion of each regularly scheduled staff meeting for continuing education. A case, or perhaps an intriguing question or two, can be ideal material for such educational sessions. For a group of people informally pursuing a single case each time they get together, the *Casebook* can be a source of productive discussion material for many months.

Supervisory Development Classes

Depending on how supervisory development classes are structured, the *Casebook* may be used either as a primary reference or as a supplement to other material. It would most appropriately be used to back up a basic supervisory development text or other instructor-provided material. Cases help bring a topic to life by moving it out of the realm of pure recitation of principles and putting it into a form in which the principles are seen in simulated action. Any topic presented in the classroom setting will be all the livelier for having its principles illustrated by one or two case studies. Use the *Casebook,* then, as a source of material to stimulate discussion following lectures or other straightforward informational presentations.

ONE TOOL IN THE TRAINING KIT

No single reference is going to be "all you ever need" for supervisory training. Similarly, no single approach to education, including the case-study approach, ever serves all purposes or fills all needs.

Any educational activity undertaken should employ a mix of available resources and materials. Even independent self-study is aided by the use of multiple viewpoints on the same topics and the presentation of the same principles in various forms and guises. In addition to providing varying perspectives on a topic, presentation variety also helps to sustain interest and involvement. Even a lone supervisor independently pursuing knowledge of, for instance, the topic of delegation, might consider using:

- a chapter on delegation from a basic text in health care supervision;
- a journal article or two concerned with delegation;
- two or three delegation cases from the *Casebook*;
- a videotape or audiotape presentation on delegation.

Independent study is always beneficial. However, group activity has the special advantages of shared insight, shared opinion, more and broader perspectives, and new ideas which are generated as participants' comments stimulate the thoughts and further comments of others. The dynamics of the group situation usually assure that the educational accomplishments of the group are greater than the direct sum of the contributions of its individual members.

In any group training activity it is important to employ a considerable mix of training approaches and instructional media. We have long accepted lectures supported by information on chalkboards, flip charts, and slides or transparencies. Although we remember but a small portion of what we simply hear, we are likely to recall a larger portion of what we see and a still larger portion of what we both see and hear. Thus a few simple visual aids to support a lecture will increase the listeners' chances of retaining more of the material.

Likewise, other training aids such as films, audiotapes, videotapes, exercises, games, and cases are all helpful when used with each other and with other forms of presentation in a healthy balance. However, no single method of instruction can be effectively employed by itself for long periods of time. Who likes to sit through two hours of lecture, without a single break in pace or manner of presentation? Who can get a great deal out of a class that consists entirely of a one-hour film? (The problems of filmed presentations are pertinent to many health care supervisors. Supervisory training usually takes place during or after working hours on at least normally hectic days, and for many folks the darkened room and the hum of the projector are invitations to dreamland.)

Many high-quality educational programs are also available on videotape or audiotape, but these too have their limitations. Even the most carefully packaged material raises questions, and it is difficult to discuss anything with a tape cassette.

An intelligent approach to supervisory development suggests that a mix of media and methods may be used to best effect in approaching a topic from numerous angles and sustaining interest through variety of presentation. Recognizing the reality of many training budgets we may not always be able to lay hands on films, tapes, and slide packages, but we can always support oral instruction with chalkboards, flip charts, and transparencies while keeping straight lecture to a tolerable minimum by using group activities such as question-and-answer sessions, learning games, exercises, role-plays, and case studies.

The case-study method is valuable; it is especially helpful in that it often stimulates further learning. It remains, however, but *one* of the training tools available to be used in combination for maximum effect.

THE NATURE OF THE CASE-STUDY APPROACH

As you go through the *Casebook* it will often seem to you that there are few absolute, specific solutions to the cases. In fact, the frequent presence of numerous implications and a variety of potential solutions is partly why group effort is especially productive in working with cases.

The *Casebook* does not include "answers" for the cases and questions because so few absolute answers are possible. Some problems may be "solved" in several different ways—all of them appropriate—depending on differences in the people involved and differences in organization policy, philosophy of operation, and the environment in which the situations occur. Most of the cases involve relations among people, and we should all be well aware that any so-called rules for dealing with people are riddled with exceptions.

In some of the cases presented, certain management fundamentals or basic principles, such as fair and equal treatment of employees, may be self-evident. Also, in some instances what is "right" or "wrong" may be obvious. However, many supposed "solutions" to case studies will take forms such as "What *might* happen if I do this?" or "I'll take this action, and if this particular result occurs I'll proceed to try this other possible step." Or simply, "This might work, or at least it seems fair and makes sense."

It should be evident to most working supervisors that there are few fixed solutions to many supervision problems. Frustrating as it seems, the correct solution to a given problem involving one employee may not be correct should a different employee be involved. If you have a dozen employees in your group you may find that on any given day there can be as many as 12 "right" ways of dealing with employees on a particular issue. As supervisors we may strive to be consistent in our application of principles and our treatment of employees as individuals. However, the employees of a department are likely to be anything but consistent in their responses to the supervisor's actions.

In management development activities, cases can help bridge the gap between theory and practice. Recognize, however, that in matters of actual practice a case is but a simulation; it is not a real problem involving real people, and it especially lacks the actual emotional involvement that a supervisor experiences with a real problem. Nevertheless, the case study represents a giant step away from theory and toward matters of practice. A primary purpose of the case method is to encourage the development and exploration of alternatives. The principal benefits of the case-study method lie not in the identification of answers but in the development of insights.

Chapter 2

The Supervisor's Essential Qualities: All Two of Them

ONLY TWO?

Yes, only two. Two particular human characteristics—and the balance between these characteristics—seem to have a major influence on whether an individual supervisor functions as a truly effective supervisor.

Recognize that we are treading on thin ice when we start talking about the characteristics of an effective supervisor, or, for that matter, the characteristics of an effective anybody. Generally the effective supervisor defies characterization; you can develop an impressive list of characteristics desirable in a supervisor and yet observe many truly effective supervisors completely lacking most of the so-called desirable characteristics.

We are not talking about job knowledge or about decision-making ability, analytical ability, the ability to delegate, the ability to use time to greatest effect, or the application of any other of the so-called management skills. Rather, we are speaking of two human characteristics which might sometimes be described as facets of personality: courage and compassion.

Regardless of knowledge of a particular working specialty or of various management techniques, in the last analysis the effective supervisor will be the person who approaches the job with the appropriate blend of courage and compassion. More than any other personal characteristics, courage and compassion, and especially the balance between them at any given time, determine how successful we are in managing the activities of other people. In short, the effective supervisor must possess the compassion to ascertain what is right under any circumstances and the courage to do what must be done.

COURAGE

Lack of courage is displayed in numerous supervisory weaknesses. It is shown, for instance, when a supervisor fails to deliver deserved criticism or so waters it down that it is ineffective simply because he or she is afraid of causing hurt, anger, frustration, or disappointment in another person. Some supervisors go to great lengths to convince themselves and others that they are not being "soft," but rather are humane and considerate. However, it is more likely that the soft supervisor is simply afraid—especially afraid of not being liked.

This same lack of courage often causes some supervisors to dilute deserved disciplinary action or avoid it altogether. Others attempt to blame the "bad stuff" on someone else. ("I want you to know this isn't my idea. *They* made me do it.") Problems get avoided or dealt with lightly and responsibilities are shirked because a soft supervisor is working hard—usually quite unconsciously—to maintain the "nice guy" image. The supervisor behaves as though evaluating every possible action and every potential decision with one question in mind: If I do it this way, will people like me less?

Granted it doesn't feel good to be put in a position of having to do something that someone else would rather you did not do. Certainly it doesn't feel good to be the one who has to step on someone's toes (although few people get their toes stepped on unless they're standing still or sitting down on the job). In some ways we may admire fictional villains, but few of us like to play the villain in real life. Given the choice, most people would rather be liked than disliked.

The effective supervisor finds it necessary to step on some toes now and then. There are, however, right and wrong ways of doing the stepping. An old bit of fortune-cookie wisdom suggests that a good supervisor is one who can step on your toes without spoiling the shine on your shoes. The supervisor needs the courage to step when stepping is necessary and the compassion to know just when, where, and how hard to step.

No doubt some managers seem to care not at all what people think of them. They seem absolutely fearless where other people's responses to their actions are concerned. However, true courage in a supervisor is not displayed by ranting and raving and pushing people around. This behavior is more indicative of plain nerve than of courage, nerve coupled with a lack of sensitivity to the feelings and needs of other people. A supervisor operating on an oversupply of brass and an undersupply of compassion charges forward with a damn-the-torpedoes attitude far more typical of a pusher than a true leader. Such behavior may represent bossism—or call it authoritarian leadership—but it does not represent effective supervision. The supervisor with real courage does not back away from certain tasks because they are difficult or unpleasant, but neither does the courageous supervisor charge boldly forward with little or no concern for people.

COMPASSION

Just as boldness and aggressiveness are often put forth as substitutes for courage, compassion also has its misapplications. Too often compassion is used as a shield for ineffectiveness, an excuse for failing to take appropriate supervisory action when called for. "Sure, maybe I was a little soft on him," says the supervisor. "I know he's been a pain in the neck, but the guy really needs the job. I know *I'd* hate to be out on the street at his age." Compassionate? Perhaps—and perhaps not. It is just as likely that the supervisor's attitude stems not from compassion, but rather from cowardice.

Backing away from tough situations is sometimes the better part of valor. However, backing away gets to be a habit for some. The truly effective supervisor will back away as far as compassion dictates, but will act with courage when the real crunch comes. The supervisor using compassion as a shield for cowardice will continue backing away beyond any reasonable point at which action should have been taken.

In the long run, the supervisor who acts out of fear of being disliked is in for a great deal of grief. Too many supervisors have discovered that no matter what they do it is not possible to be liked by everyone. It is far better to strive to acquire the respect of your employees. A person's respect can be earned through fair and impartial dealings and held by maintaining the relationship on the same level. On the other hand, a person's affection must be earned all over again each time a hurdle in the relationship is approached.

Compassion, of course, is caring, caring for patients, employees, visitors, and others. Compassion does not consist of timid behavior in the face of potential anger or displeasure. It involves treating all people with dignity and respect, and being polite, considerate, and generally humane with all persons, even those who have broken the rules. The compassionate supervisor also knows that more may be accomplished with reason and understanding than with anger or force.

THE BALANCING ACT

Part of the difficulty in striking—or, for that matter, even describing—the appropriate balance between courage and compassion lies in widespread differences in human understanding of these characteristics. Courage and compassion simply do not rate equally with everyone.

To most people courage is a good word; it has a bold, brave sound to it. It describes a noble and desirable characteristic, and most people believe it is admirable to be considered courageous. Compassion, however, is another matter. While compassion is a positive word for most people, it nevertheless does not rate as highly as courage.

The human relations movement in management is largely a product of the middle part of the twentieth century. Years ago, compassion had little place in organized work activity. Many employees had no voice in how they did their work; they did as they were told, or they sought work elsewhere. A boss was a boss, and a worker was a worker, and the boss was always right.

Old, widespread notions change slowly and with great difficulty. For more than a few people the word "compassion" continues to suggest a degree of weakness, and few of us wish to be considered weak in any respect. True compassion, however, is not weakness, any more than simple boldness is courage.

In addition to seeing shades of weakness in compassion, some supervisors also see many of their employees as not truly deserving their compassion. A supervisor's perspective often becomes distorted by repeated dealings with the same people week in and week out. Just as a police officer may sometimes develop a negative outlook by dealing with the same small but troublesome element of society day after day, the supervisor may similarly develop a negative attitude. After all, a large part of a supervisor's life consists of dealing with employees face to face and solving problems which spring from employees' behavior. It is the chronic misbehavers, usually a small percentage of the work force, who the supervisor sees and becomes aware of most.

The capacity for compassion suffers as the negative attitude toward people grows. Some supervisors come to believe that management is less "getting things done through people" than it is getting things done *in spite of* people.

The supervisor has a job to do. That job consists largely of getting other jobs, perhaps a great many of them, done through the efforts of other people. Doing this effectively requires that the supervisor exercise compassion in recognizing and treating each employee as an individual and at the same time exercise sufficient courage to keep employees' efforts channeled toward fulfillment of the goals of the organization. Whether practicing supervision at the workplace or attempting to develop one's supervisory skills further—for instance, in considering the cases and questions in the *Casebook*—the effective supervisor will be the one who exhibits the courage necessary to do what must be done and the compassion to get it done with every human consideration.

Chapter 3

The Emphasis: Determining What's Important to the Supervisor

BACKGROUND

A Look at Needs

In the mid-1970s a committee of health facility administrators, personnel directors, training managers, and management development instructors was charged with developing a course in basic supervisory skills for health care supervisors. Drawn from the membership of an association of hospitals and other health facilities, the committee was to determine what topics the course should include and the emphasis to be placed on each topic. The association intended to make the course available to any of the association's member institutions that wished to use it, and to offer it later for use by institutions in other areas.

Most of the committee members had previous experience with management development programs, and although they all had some fairly definite ideas of what such a program should include they had little difficulty reaching agreement on the recommended contents of the course.

Topic emphasis, on the other hand, was quite another matter. There was only partial agreement among committee members as to which topics should be stressed for any particular group of supervisors. Except for citing a few obvious common topic areas (decision making and face-to-face communication, for instance) the committee did not achieve substantial agreement in dealing with the question of which topics were more important to the majority of supervisors most of the time.

The committee felt that the dozen topic areas they had identified suggested the arrangement of material by topic modules. That is, a dozen topics could be organized into 12 distinctly different modules, each of which could be presented as a single class. However, the committee, working with the association's member institutions, had also decided that eight classes was the practical maximum course length. The majority of institutions surveyed on the possible combinations of class length and number of classes expressed a preference for a series of eight two-hour classes, one class each week for eight weeks.

There seemed to be but two choices: Build the supervisory skills course around eight of the committee's twelve topics while saving the other four for a possible follow-up program; or compress some of the topics to present all twelve within eight classes. But which topics should be left out of the basic course, or which should be compressed? The committee could come up with no generally acceptable answers to this question. The following statement summarizes the committee's position:

> The limitations presented by eight two-hour sessions allow little time in which to provide an effective orientation to supervision. Indeed, even with twice that amount of time we could do little more than scratch the surface of some of the important topics. Moreover, it is likely that the needs of any particular group of supervisors taking the course will be different from the needs of other groups. We would like to be able to present a course which is sufficiently flexible to meet the needs of any particular group; for instance, a program covering all 12 topics but in which the instructors can emphasize certain topics as the needs of the group emerge.

A tentative order of the topics was established, but, except for designating a module concerning basic management fundamentals as the opening session, little attention was given to topic order. The matter of topic emphasis was left open; in the opening session of each course the supervisors in the class would help the instructor determine their own topic emphasis.

The Topics

The following are brief descriptions of the 12 topic modules outlined by the committee, listed in the order in which they appeared in the tentative course outline given to the first few class groups.

 1. *The Management Process.* Introduction to the fundamentals of management; the basic management functions—planning, organizing, directing, coordinating, and controlling; the supervisor's two roles—worker and manager; management as "getting things done through people."

2. *Written Communication.* The basics of effective writing on the job; effective letters, memoranda, and brief reports; taking the agony out of everyday writing.
3. *Group Communication.* Meetings—their advantages and disadvantages; types of meetings and their uses; conducting effective meetings.
4. *Change.* Resistance to change—how and why it develops; how to recognize and deal with resistance; how to head it off before it can develop.
5. *Decision Making.* The elements of the basic decision-making process; risk, uncertainty, and judgment; when to decide—and when to decide not to decide.
6. *One-to-One Communication.* The face-to-face nature of the supervisory task; the supervisor-employee relationship; barriers to effective interpersonal communication and how to avoid them; effective listening.
7. *Employee Motivation.* Finding out what makes people perform; the motivators and the dissatisfiers; some steps toward true motivation.
8. *Delegation.* The importance of delegation in getting things done through people; how to bring person and task together for effective delegation; delegation as a key to supervisory effectiveness.
9. *Personal Supervisory Effectiveness.* Time management—the supervisor versus the clock; personal organization; planning and the establishment of priorities.
10. *Creativity.* The role of creativity in everyday problem solving and decision making; the elements of creativity; generating ideas when none are apparent.
11. *Methods Improvement.* Improved departmental effectiveness through improved work methods; analyzing and improving work methods; working smarter, not harder.
12. *Unionization.* Union organizing—the signs and signals; the supervisor's key role during a union organizing drive; living and dealing with a union.

The Topic Survey

Beginning with the first group to assemble for the supervisory skills course, the attendees received a survey form listing the titles and descriptions of the 12 topic areas. Following a brief oral expansion of the topic descriptions and a question-and-answer session, the attendees rated the topics according to their personal needs for knowledge on their jobs. In effect, the supervisors were responding to this question: What is the order of importance of these topics to *you* in your supervisory position?

Several class groups successfully determined the topic emphasis using this simple survey. The process, however, was cumbersome; although the supervisors needed only a few minutes to establish their topic rankings, it took about 30 minutes to tabulate the rankings and establish an average order of emphasis for a group of 25 supervisors. Also, the judgmental difficulties involved in "sorting out" a number of impressions at the same time—much like juggling 12 oranges at once—suggested that the results left something to be desired even when assessing something as abstract as individual perceptions of needs.

Nevertheless, useful information was gained from the topic surveys, and the early courses, presented with the groups' self-determined needs in mind, were well attended and marked by high levels of attendee participation. So course instructors considered ways to conduct the topic survey that would make the results more useful. The method selected involved the use of analysis by *forced-choice pairs*.

Described in detail in the remainder of this chapter, analysis by forced-choice pairs is a technique highly applicable to the establishment of rankings when the topics or items to be ranked cannot be measured objectively. The process allows us to sort out our judgments by systematically comparing each item to every other item one at a time.

At this stage of the discussion the notion of the topic survey is fully as important as the 12 topic areas going into the original supervisory skills course. The topic survey has been applied successfully for several years in establishing the topic emphasis for new programs as well as for determining topic emphasis for individual supervisory skills class groups. Further, much of the emphasis of the material in this book—the topics of the cases, problems, and questions used—was determined by what numerous supervisors said, through their topic surveys, about matters of concern to them.

Admittedly the foregoing lies in the past, but the topic survey approach can prove valuable in many applications well beyond these pages. The method of forced-choice pairs can be used to generate a relative ranking of any set of factors or characteristics which do not lend themselves to measurement in any quantitative sense. More specifically, it can help you assess learning needs and prepare for any management development activity.

If you happen to be an administrator, personnel or training director, or management development instructor, using the forced-choice pairs method with your own list of topics can give you a solid idea of learning needs as perceived by any group of actual or potential course attendees. Based on what you learn you can either include or exclude certain topics, devote more time to some topics and less to others, or establish a preferred order of topic presentation.

If you are an individual supervisor using this volume out of personal interest, you can learn a great deal about your management development needs relative to your job. Initially, try going through the foregoing list of topics using the method of forced-choice pairs. Each time you look at a pair of topics ask yourself: Of these two areas of management skill, which one is more important to me most of the time? As suggested earlier, it is difficult to separate judgmentally a dozen factors from each other all at the same time. The forced-choice pairs method allows you to reduce what is essentially a gross judgment call to a series of independent, one-on-one judgments which can later be tabulated to arrive at an overall tendency. Even if you believe you already have a clear picture of your job needs, you may still be in for a surprise or two.

FORCED-CHOICE PAIRS, APPLIED

A person asked to "sort out" the foregoing 12 topics would first be given a form much like Exhibit 3–1. On the form each number is paired once with every other number. The top row in the triangular pattern of pairs always contains one pair less than the number of items involved. In this case there are 11 pairs in the first row because number 1 is paired, in turn, with 2 through 12. Each succeeding row is shorter by one pair than the previous row. For example, the second row starts with 2; there is no need to pair 2 with 1 in this row, since that was already done in the first row. There are 11 rows in all.

There are 66 pairs in the matrix $(11 + 10 + 9 + 8 + 7 + 6 + 5 + 4 + 3 + 2 + 1)$, so 66 choices must be accounted for in the tabulation.

Using the matrix of pairs essentially amounts to asking yourself 66 similar questions. For instance, the first question, the choice between number 1 and number two, is: Which is *more* important to me *most* of the time, knowledge of the management process (#1) or knowledge of written communication (#2)? In this manner each choice is made free of all other considerations and each result is preserved for later use.

Now look at Exhibit 3–2, the same matrix as it might be used by someone rating our 12 supervisory skills topics. A simple tabulation captures the number of times each topic was chosen and allows us to account for all 66 choices. The tabulation also shows the order of emphasis resulting from this particular set of choices.

Considering the results of the tabulation in Exhibit 3–2, you may wonder about the presence of a couple of apparent ties: #2 and #3 are tied at five each and account for positions 6 and 7; #1 and #4 are tied at four each

Exhibit 3-1 Matrix of Pairs for Twelve Items

1	1	1	1	1	1	1	1	1	1	1
2	3	4	5	6	7	8	9	10	11	12
	2	2	2	2	2	2	2	2	2	2
	3	4	5	6	7	8	9	10	11	12
		3	3	3	3	3	3	3	3	3
		4	5	6	7	8	9	10	11	12
			4	4	4	4	4	4	4	4
			5	6	7	8	9	10	11	12
				5	5	5	5	5	5	5
				6	7	8	9	10	11	12
					6	6	6	6	6	6
					7	8	9	10	11	12
						7	7	7	7	7
						8	9	10	11	12
							8	8	8	8
							9	10	11	12
								9	9	9
								10	11	12
									10	10
									11	12
										11
										12

and account for positions 8 and 9. However, these are not really exact ties. Any two tied numbers can be separated by considering which of them won the individual choice over the other. Thus in Exhibit 3-2, #2 takes position 6, #3 takes position 7, #4 takes position 8, and #1 is left with position 9. You are left with a clear order of preference.

What if you have a three-way tie, or even a four-way tie? Simply take the tied items and set them up in a small matrix of pairs of their own. Exhibit 3-3 assumes a four-way tie among items 5, 7, 8, and 9, covering positions 2, 3, 4, and 5. Should two-way ties occur in this small "runoff," they are easily resolved as previously described.

Exhibit 3-4 is the analysis of Exhibit 3-2 with the two-way ties resolved and additional information provided. The "Divided by 66" column, in which each calculation has the effect of saying what fractional part of 66 that number's selections accounted for, is the first step in creating the

Exhibit 3–2 Rating: Twelve Topics

```
①  1   1   1   1   1   1   1   ①   ①   ①
2   ③   ④   ⑤   ⑥   ⑦   ⑧   ⑨  10  11  12
    ②   ②   2   2   2   2   2   ②   ②   ②
    3   4   ⑤   ⑥   ⑦   ⑧   ⑨  10  11  12
        ③   3   3   3   3   3   ③   ③   ③
        4   ⑤   ⑥   ⑦   ⑧   ⑨  10  11  12
            4   4   4   4   4   ④   ④   ④
            ⑤   ⑥   ⑦   ⑧   ⑨  10  11  12
                5   ⑤   ⑤   ⑤   ⑤   ⑤   ⑤
                ⑥   7   8   9  10  11  12
                    ⑥   ⑥   ⑥   ⑥   ⑥   ⑥
                    7   8   9  10  11  12
                        7   ⑦   ⑦   ⑦   ⑦
                        ⑧   9  10  11  12
                            ⑧   ⑧   ⑧   ⑧
                            9  10  11  12
                                ⑨   ⑨   ⑨
                                10  11  12
                                    ⑩   ⑩
                                    11  12
                                        ⑪
                                        12
```

Number of:		Order
1s	4	8,9
2s	5	6,7
3s	5	6,7
4s	4	8,9
5s	10	2
6s	11	1
7s	8	4
8s	9	3
9s	7	5
10s	2	10
11s	1	11
12s	0	12
	66	

Exhibit 3–3 Tie-Breaking Rating: Four Items

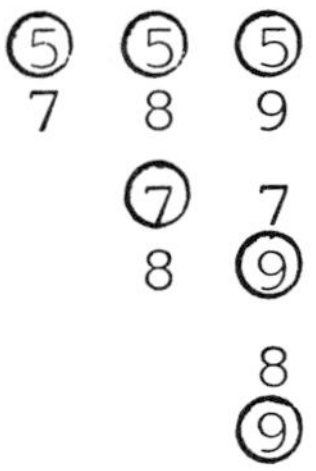

```
Number of 5s = 3, so #5 takes position 2.

Number of 7s = 1, so #7 takes position 4.

Number of 8s = 0, so #8 takes position 5.

Number of 9s = 2, so #9 takes position 3.
```

"Index." The index numbers come about when each decimal in the "Divided by 66" column is subsequently divided by the largest decimal in the column. Thus the item that ranks first in order has an index of 1.00, and all the others are scaled relative to the number-one choice.

The effect of the index is to provide an idea of the importance of any individual item relative to the "most important" item (number one in "Order"). For instance, in Exhibit 3–4, the evaluator considered topic #4—in eighth position with an index of 0.35—to be roughly one-third as important as topic #6 (in first position, with index 1.00). Similarly, topic #1 (ninth position, index 0.35) was considered about half as important as topic #7 (fourth position, index 0.71).

The point of the foregoing discussion is twofold. In addition to introducing the technique of forced-choice pairs, a method of ranking items which cannot be measured objectively, it also lays the groundwork for the introduction of a comprehensive learning-needs survey which can now be described.

SUPERVISORY TOPIC-PREFERENCE SURVEY

For about three and one-half years, each group of supervisors starting the course described at the beginning of this chapter was surveyed using the forced-choice pairs method. There were 45 groups, each consisting of 18 to 25 working health care supervisors. Average group size was 22; all

Exhibit 3–4 Rating and Ranking: Twelve Topics

Paired-comparison chart (circled number = selected in each pair):

Row 1: ①/2 1/③ 1/④ 1/⑤ 1/⑥ 1/⑦ 1/⑧ 1/⑨ ①/10 ①/11 ①/12
Row 2: ②/3 ②/4 2/⑤ 2/⑥ 2/⑦ 2/⑧ 2/⑨ ②/10 ②/11 ②/12
Row 3: ③/4 3/⑤ 3/⑥ 3/⑦ 3/⑧ 3/⑨ ③/10 ③/11 ③/12
Row 4: 4/⑤ 4/⑥ 4/⑦ 4/⑧ 4/⑨ ④/10 ④/11 ④/12
Row 5: 5/⑥ ⑤/7 ⑤/8 ⑤/9 ⑤/10 ⑤/11 ⑤/12
Row 6: ⑥/7 ⑥/8 ⑥/9 ⑥/10 ⑥/11 ⑥/12
Row 7: 7/⑧ ⑦/9 ⑦/10 ⑦/11 ⑦/12
Row 8: ⑧/9 ⑧/10 ⑧/11 ⑧/12
Row 9: ⑨/10 ⑨/11 ⑨/12
Row 10: ⑩/11 ⑩/12
Row 11: ⑪/12

Number of:		Divided by 66	Index	Order
1s	4	0.06	0.35	9
2s	5	0.08	0.47	6
3s	5	0.08	0.47	7
4s	4	0.06	0.35	8
5s	10	0.15	0.88	2
6s	11	0.17	1.00	1
7s	8	0.12	0.71	4
8s	9	0.14	0.82	3
9s	7	0.11	0.65	5
10s	2	0.03	0.18	10
11s	1	0.02	0.12	11
12s	0	0	0	12
	66	1.00		

in all, the 45 groups totaled 990 supervisors. These 990 supervisors were employees of 36 institutions, 34 hospitals and 2 nursing homes. In some instances, several small hospitals shared classes. Some large hospitals ran multiple classes for different groups of supervisors.

Each supervisor rated the topics, and the ratings of all supervisors in each group were combined for a group rating. Eventually the ratings of the 45 groups were combined. The results of the combination appear in Exhibit 3–5.

Exhibit 3–5 lists the 12 topics in rank order. An index number is shown for each as an approximation of the relative importance of each topic. Primarily this list tells us that for a particular population of supervisors— 990 supervisors from 36 institutions—this is the average order of importance of the topics.

While One-to-One Communication (#6) ranked first, Decision Making (#5) and Employee Motivation (#7) were so close as to be considered fully as important (index numbers 0.94 and 0.90). Indeed, any basic supervisory program that concentrates on these three topics cannot help but be relevant to many attendees, and it was precisely on this basis that a new first-level supervisory program was developed. In structuring this new program, the topic preference of Exhibit 3–5 was altered in just one way: the treatment of resistance to change (Change, ranked eighth). Overcoming employee resistance to change appeared to pose problems related largely to one-to-one communication and motivation, so *Change* was incorporated into the new first-level program.

A second-level program soon followed, built primarily around Delegation and other aspects of Personal Supervisory Effectiveness.

Exhibit 3–5 Summary Ranking: 45 Groups, 990 Supervisors

Topic	Index	Rank
(#6) One-to-One Communication	1.00	1
(#5) Decision Making	0.94	2
(#7) Employee Motivation	0.90	3
(#8) Delegation	0.74	4
(#9) Personal Supervisory Effectiveness	0.70	5
(#1) The Management Process	0.69	6
(#3) Group Communication	0.67	7
(#4) Change	0.66	8
(#2) Written Communication	0.56	9
(#11) Methods Improvement	0.54	10
(#10) Creativity	0.53	11
(#12) Unionization	0.37	12

Separate programs and seminars, later offered on an as-needed or as-desired basis, were developed for conference leadership (Group Communication), effective writing (Written Communication), creative problem solving (Creativity), labor relations (Unionization), and Methods Improvement. This approach recognized that some topics that might not be high on a supervisor's list of needs in general, for example unionization, were nevertheless quite important to some supervisors some of the time.

CASEBOOK TOPIC EMPHASIS

The topic-preference survey just described was tempered with experience to create the topic emphasis of this book. Although the *Casebook* employs relatively simple breakdowns (see Chapter 4, "Introduction to Cases," and Chapter 8, "Introduction to Questions"), these breakdowns stress the topic areas highlighted by the topic-preference survey. For instance, because most supervisors said via surveys and classroom comments that most of their problems involved communications (primarily with employees, sometimes with superiors, and occasionally with peers), the *Casebook* devotes considerable attention to communications problems—mostly with employees.

It is important to recognize that few, if any, of the topic areas so far discussed are mutually exclusive. For instance, consideration of delegation is consideration of a "skill' or a "technique," but active delegation poses problems in communication, decision making, motivation, and other areas. Also, consideration of some of the topics opens other areas not listed and not yet considered but still deserving mention. Many of the problems of employee communication, for example, eventually involve criticism and discipline, leading us to consider organizational characteristics, such as rules and policies, and concepts such as authority.

If, however, you were to screen the contents of the *Casebook* carefully and arrange them according to the rankings of Exhibit 3–5 you would discover that the generic topic areas receiving the most attention are those near the top of the list. Quite simply, the *Casebook* places most emphasis on those topics that seem to mean the most to working health care supervisors.

Chapter 4

Introduction to Cases

THREE VIEWS OF THE SUPERVISOR'S JOB

In examining the kinds of problems you face as a supervisor it is helpful to consider the supervisory job from three points of view: the people you must deal with; the task you must perform; and the effectiveness with which you must apply yourself. Most supervisory problems involve some mix of all three—people, task, and self—but depending on the nature of a particular problem some of these are more likely to be involved than others.

It is generally recognized—and certainly recognized throughout the *Casebook*—that the majority of supervisors' problems are people problems. Most of these people problems, in turn, seem to involve employees, and the next greatest number involve superiors, usually a supervisor's immediate manager. Other people problems are likely to involve peers as well as the employees and superiors of other supervisors. Indeed, many difficulties that are often thought of as "organizational problems" are actually people problems, since an organization and its functioning consists largely of the organization's members and their interactions.

People problems bring into play all topics that are in any way relevant to interpersonal relations. These pertinent topics include:

- communication of all kinds and in all organizational directions;
- criticism and discipline, the application of specific approaches to particular kinds of people problems;
- leadership, and dealing with human responses to various leadership styles;

- motivation, including people's varying needs and their differing responses to diverse forces and pressures; and
- numerous other topics that have their foundations in various aspects of human behavior.

In short, the people viewpoint broadly encompasses all supervisory job elements that involve relations with people.

The task view of the supervisory job focuses on things the supervisor must *do*, on techniques that must be practiced in the process of getting things done through people. Topics with a strong task orientation include the management of change, decision making, the application of basic management principles, the practice of labor relations, the improvement of work methods, the conduct of meetings, etc.

Although one or the other may dominate in any given situation, the people and task aspects of the supervisor's job are interrelated. Never completely separable, the manner in which each is pursued affects the other. Consider, for example, the practice of decision making. Decision making poorly practiced, where the solution is ill-conceived, arbitrary, and poorly communicated, will inevitably cause more people problems, but decision making skillfully practiced with all human consideration can minimize resulting people problems. Thus the task and its performance and people and how they are dealt with, while representing different views of the supervisory role, have a constant and undeniable influence on each other.

The line between the task and self views of the supervisor's job might at times seem to be so finely drawn as to be nearly undetectable. The distinction, however, is helpful in allowing us to consider certain aspects of the supervisor's job that are most strongly related to personal approach and performance. Under self we are primarily considering supervisors as managers of themselves in allocating time, setting priorities, and taking various other steps to assure personal effectiveness. Some self-related activities, such as time management and personal organization, appear much like task-related activities in that they call upon supervisors to put particular techniques into practice. Others, delegation foremost among them, seem to involve important dealings with people as well as the application of management techniques. The major emphasis, however, of delegation, time management, and other aspects of the practice of personal effectiveness is the management of self *by* self.

The three views of the supervisor's job—people, task, and self—thus briefly describe the things you have to do as a supervisor: Manage (or relate to, or get along with) *people;* manage the *task* through the application of various techniques; and manage *yourself.*

These three views became the first level of classification for arranging material for the *Casebook*. This first-level classification, or primary focus, identifies the preferred viewpoint from which a particular case should initially be examined. Thus the primary focus is suggesting that a case should be viewed primarily in one of three ways:

- as a problem with people and how to work with them and relate to them;
- as a problem with the supervisory task and how various management concepts and techniques are applied;
- as a problem with self, or how the supervisor personally approaches the job.

Any topic relevant to supervision, and certainly any particular case in the *Casebook,* may be viewed in more than one way. Consider, for instance, a case concerned with the topic of delegation, keeping in mind the earlier suggestion that how well a supervisor delegates may be considered a measure of how well that supervisor manages *self*. A specific case on delegation may have either people, task, or self as its primary focus. Perhaps the focus is on people because the major difficulty in the case involves an employee's reluctance to accept responsibility or exercise delegated authority. Perhaps the case focuses on task, concentrating on preparing the instructions or making the decisions necessary to pave the way for actual delegation. Or the focus may be on self, on how thoroughly the supervisor accepts the necessity of delegation and determines to apply it as a way of improving personal effectiveness.

CLASSIFICATION OF CASES

Each case appearing in Chapter 5 is identified according to four categories of information:

1. *Primary Focus.* In some instances an obvious designation, in others an arbitrary assignment, the primary focus targets the most potentially productive viewpoint—people, task, or self—for initial consideration of the case.
2. *Secondary Focus.* The secondary focus calls attention to another pertinent, although perhaps somewhat subordinate, viewpoint from which the case may be examined. For instance, a case heading identifying people as the primary focus and self as the secondary focus is in effect telling you: This is first and foremost a case involving

people problems, but it is also worth considering as a case in how you handle yourself as supervisor.

3. *Topic Emphasis.* The next level of breakdown beneath focus, this highlights the principal topic of the case. There are a number of possible topics, including many of those introduced in Chapter 3 as well as several additional topics. For instance, a case whose principal topic is change management, whether its primary focus was, for instance, people or task, deals with some aspect of change, whether this be planning for a change, evaluating a potential change, or working to overcome resistance to change.

4. *Additional Topics.* Identified under this heading are other pertinent topics for which the case will provide food for thought. At least two, and in most instances three, additional topics are indicated for each case. This tells you simply that a particular case is applicable in the consideration of certain topics other than the major topic of the case.

THE *CASEBOOK* EMPHASIS

The problems and questions offered by numerous supervisors, plus the general direction indicated by the topic-preference survey detailed in Chapter 3, suggest that most supervisors rate the three views of the supervisor's job in this order: people first; task second; and self third. The cases appearing in Chapter 5 (as well as the questions utilized in Chapter 9) were assembled according to this order of importance.

People appears as the primary focus of more than 70 percent of the cases in Chapter 5. All together, 90 percent of the cases have *people* as either the primary or the secondary focus; in 88 percent of the cases *task* is either the primary or the secondary focus (in most instances in which *people* is the primary focus, *task* is the secondary focus). Cases in which *self* is either the primary or the secondary focus amount to about 14 percent of the total.

In terms of topics, *communication* is either the major topic or an additional topic in 85 percent of the cases. In fact, there are very few cases that do not have clear communications implications—reflecting the strong concern of most supervisors for the importance of one-to-one communication in the performance of their jobs.

TOPIC NUMBERING AND CROSS-REFERENCE

Each case number begins with a prefix consisting of two capital letters divided by a slash to indicate primary and secondary focus. The letter "P" stands for people, "T" for task, and "S" for self. This is followed by a dash and a two-digit number used to identify major topic, and another dash and two-digit number to indicate the sequential number of the case within the major topic. For example, since 01 is the major topic number for change management, Case P/T–01–05 is the fifth case in change management having people as its primary focus and task as its secondary focus.

An occasional entry is further identified by a one-letter suffix in parentheses to indicate either a role-play (R) or an exercise (E) rather than a straightforward case.

The following is an alphabetical listing of topics identified in the case headings in Chapter 5 as major topics, additional topics, or both.

Topic	Major topic of:	Additional topic of:
(01) Change Management	P/T–01–01, –02, –03, –04 T/P–01–01, –02, –03, –04, –05 T/S–01–01 (E)	P/T–02–01; –05–01 (R); –13–01; –16–01 T/P–11–01, –02, –03 S/T–14–01, –02
(02) Communication	P/T–02–01, –02, –03, –04, –05, –06 (E), –07 P/S–02–01 (R), –02	P/T–01–01, –02, –03, –04; –03–01, –02 (R), –03, –04, –05, –06; –05–01 (R), –02, –03, –04, –05; 07–01, –02; –08–02; –09–01; –13–01, –02, –03, –04, –05, –06, –07, –08, –10, –11, –12; –15–01 (R), –02, –03, –04 (R), –05; –16–02, –03, –04, –05, –06, –07, –08 (R) P/S–05–01, –02; –13–01; –16–01; –17–01 T/P–01–01, –02, –03, –04, –05; –04–01;

Topic	Major topic of:	Additional topic of:
		−07−01 (E); −10−01; −11−01, −02
		T/S−06−01, −02, −03
		S/P−05−01; −14−01
		S/T−14−01, −03, −04
(03) Criticism and Discipline	P/T−03−01, −02 (R), −03, −04, −05, −06	P/T−13−02, −03, −04; −16−02, −03, −04
		P/S−02−01 (R); −13−01
(04) Decision Making	T/P−04−01	P/T−08−01, −02; −13−01, −05, −06, −09; −16−01, −02, −05
		T/P−01−01; −11−03
		S/T−14−02
(05) Delegation	P/T−05−01 (R), −02, −03, −04, −05	P/T−02−02; −03−01; −13−07; −16−06
	P/S−05−01, −02	P/S−02−02; −13−01
	S/P−05−01	
	S/T−05−01	
(06) General Management Practice	T/S−06−01, −02, −03	P/T−02−02
		S/T−05−01
(07) Hiring	P/T−07−01, −02	P/T−03−02 (R); −16−03
	T/P−07−01 (E)	
(08) Labor Relations	P/T−08−01, −02	P/T−03−03
(09) Leadership	P/T−09−01	P/T−01−01, −02, −04; −02−03, −04; −03−06; −05−02; −08−02; −13−12; −15−01 (R); −16−07

		P/S–05–01; –16–01
		T/P–01–02; –11–02
		T/S–06–01
		S/P–14–01
		S/T–05–01; –14–02
(10) Meetings	T/P–10–01	P/T–01–03; –02–01, –05; –03–04
(11) Methods Improvement	T/P–11–01, –02, –03	P/T–13–08
		T/P–01–03, –04; –04–01
		T/S–01–01 (E)
(12) Motivation	(none)	P/T–01–01, –04; –02–01, –03, –06 (E), –07; –03–04, –05; –05–03, –04; –13–02, –03, –07
		P/S–05–02
		T/P–01–01, –02, –03, –05; –10–01; –11–03
		S/P–05–01
(13) People Problems	P/T–13–01, –02, –03, –04, –05, –06, –07, –08, –09, –10, –11, –12 P/S–13–01	P/T–02–03, –05, –06 (E), –07; –03–01, –05, –06; –05–03; –07–01; –15–02, –03, –04 (R), –05; –16–01, –05, –07, –08 (R)
		P/S–02–01 (R); –05–01, –02; –16–01
		T/P–01–04, –05; –04–01; –10–01
		T/S–06–02, –03

Topic	Major topic of:	Additional topic of:
(14) Personal Effectiveness	S/P–14–01 S/T–14–01, –02, –03, –04	P/T–02–04; –16–08 (R) P/S–02–01 (R), –02; –17–01 T/S–01–01 (E); –06–01, –02, –03 S/P–05–01 S/T–05–01
(15) Rules and Policies	P/T–15–01 (R), –02, –03, –04 (R), –05	P/T–03–02 (R), –03; –07–01, 02; –08–01; –13–10, –11; –16–04 T/P–07–01 (E)
(16) Supervisory Authority	P/T–16–01, –02, –03, –04, –05, –06, –07, –08 (R) P/S–16–01	P/T–01–02, –03; –02–02, –04, –05, –07; –05–01 (R), –04, –05; –07–02; –08–01; –09–01; –13–04, –06, –08, –10, –11; –15–01 (R), –03, –04 (R), –05 P/S–02–02; –17–01 T/P–07–01 (E)
(17) Time Management	P/S–17–01	S/T–14–01, –03, –04

AN EXAMPLE

Consider Case P/T–01–03 titled "It Wasn't *My* Decision." The heading of this case is:

Primary Focus:	People
Secondary Focus:	Task
Topic Emphasis:	Change Management
Additional Topics:	Communication, Meetings, Supervisory Authority

Without reading beyond the heading you know that this case focuses most strongly on people problems (primary focus) but also provides worthwhile discussion material about the application of some management concepts or techniques (secondary focus). Further, you know that the case deals largely with the management of change (topic emphasis, or major topic), and that this case may be productively employed in any discussion or other consideration of the topics of communication, meetings, and supervisory authority.

Also, you are likely to discover that when you have "opened up" some cases through reading and discussion you will identify other pertinent topics beyond those additional topics listed in the heading. For instance, Case P/T–01–03 will also appear to have implications for the topic of methods improvement when we begin to consider the mechanics of the particular systems problems involved in the case.

A SAMPLE CASE

It has already been suggested that there are few specific, absolute "answers" to most case studies in health care supervision. What works in one instance may not work at all in another, although both instances may seem nearly identical on the surface. What works with one person or a particular group of people may not work or perhaps even have negative effects if different personalities are involved.

What is correct for *you* as a supervisor may depend considerably on your personal supervisory style and the strength of your relationships with your employees, your boss, and your peers. You cannot help but bring your style and your knowledge of your relationships into your consideration of most case studies.

The suggested solution to the problem presented in a case can rarely be labeled absolutely "right" or "wrong." Rather, the suggested solution will likely possess some degree of appropriateness—or perhaps inappropriateness—depending on a multitude of factors that surround the specific incident dealt with in the case.

The relative appropriateness of your analysis of a case will, of course, be partly determined by your management knowledge and supervisory skill and how you apply this knowledge and skill. If you find you are in familiar territory, that you are properly guided by successful experience and sound knowledge of the topics involved, you may be able to zero in quite readily on a possibly workable solution. However, if you proceed with doubt, and your pursuit of the case seems to raise more questions than it answers, perhaps you need to research some information about the case topics or discuss the case with others.

The sample case discussed in the following paragraphs is taken from Group 3 in Chapter 5. It is stressed that the answers to the questions are not the only possible correct answers; they are simply one possible set of "good" answers—"good" because they are based on a number of sound management principles.

The sample case is number T/P–01–02, so the primary focus is *task* and the secondary focus is *people*. The major topic is *change management* and the most visible additional topics are *communication, leadership,* and *motivation*.

Surprise!

On Monday morning when the business office employees arrived at the hospital they immediately noticed the apparent absence of the office manager. This was not unusual; the manager was frequently absent on Monday. However, he rarely failed to call his department when he would not be there—but on this day he still had not called by noon.

Shortly after lunch the two working supervisors in the business office were summoned to the administrator's office. There they were told that the office manager was no longer employed by the hospital. They, the two supervisors, were told to look after things for the current week and that a new manager, already secured, would be starting the following Monday. All the supervisors were told about the new manager was that it was somebody from outside the hospital.

The supervisors were not told whether the former manager resigned or was discharged, nor were they told whether anyone within the department had been considered as a replacement.

Questions

  1. What was right or wrong about the manner in which the change in business office manager was made?

2. What would you suppose to be the attitudes of the business office staff upon hearing of the change?
3. With what attitudes do you suppose the staff will receive the new manager?
4. In what other ways might this change have been approached?

Responses to Questions

1. Not a great deal appears to have been right in the manner in which the change in business office manager was made. We may probably infer correctly that the former manager was fired, but there is not enough information in the case to allow us to judge whether the firing was deserved by the manager and done in the best interest of the hospital.

It was wrong for the department's staff to be left in the dark even for the half-Monday during which they drifted without knowing that the person they thought of as boss was no longer their boss. It was also wrong to announce the new manager's coming without first telling the two supervisors why they were not considered for the position.

It was, however, right for administration to avoid telling the department that the manager was leaving before the departure actually occurred. If the manager was indeed fired, the reasons for and the timing of that firing were nobody's business but the manager's and administration's. It would certainly have helped for the staff to have had time to prepare themselves for the changeover, but the apparent nature of the manager's termination did not make this possible. Thus it was probably right for administration to remain silent about the probable firing; however, it was wrong for administration to fail to take steps to make the transition as smooth as possible under the circumstances. Appropriate steps should have begun no later than first thing Monday morning.

2. The attitudes of the business office staff might vary from person to person, including:

- *relief* on the part of some who may not have fared well under the previous manager;
- *anger* and *resentment* by some who may conclude that the ever-powerful "they" (administration) had moved against one of the department's number (sometimes a firing will bring out sympathy and support where they did not previously exist);
- *disappointment,* especially on the part of the two supervisors who did not have a chance to try for the job, but also felt by others who are advancement-oriented and now see that no promotional opportunities will be opening up in the department;

- *rejection* felt by some—again, especially the two supervisors—who may feel they have been excluded from important happenings (the effect of the half-day of silence);
- *apprehension* regarding the incoming manager who remains a totally unknown quantity.

In short, the total effect on staff morale and motivation could be devastating. Especially during the week without a manager the group could be gloomy, fearful, and angry—and may produce very little real work. It could require a new manager of extraordinary leadership ability to bring the department back to its former level of productivity in a reasonable period of time.

3. The staff is likely to receive the new manager with caution and apprehension. Regardless of whether most of the staff liked or disliked the former manager, they *knew* him. They do not yet know the new manager, so they are "off balance," that is, their equilibrium has been disturbed in a manner as yet unknown to them. Regarding the past manager's departure some may think, "They got the boss, so how secure am *I*?" Indeed, some staff members may well wonder if the incoming manager will be the new broom that sweeps clean.

The presence of such attitudes may inspire intradepartmental maneuvering as people jockey for position and attempt to achieve favorable status relative to the new manager.

4. As to how the change might otherwise have been approached, the following steps might have been considered by administration:

- Assuming the former manager was released at the end of Friday, get to the two supervisors at once, ideally over the weekend but certainly no later than the start of business Monday, and tell them of the manager's departure (the fact of the departure, but not the reasons behind it).
- Spend a few minutes with each supervisor alone to tell each, in specific terms, why he or she was not being considered for the position. The supervisors deserve this consideration.
- Instruct both supervisors to conduct business as usual with their respective groups while reporting directly to administration for that week only.
- Tell the supervisors about the incoming manager—name, background, experience, etc.—to help reduce the unknowns about the yet-to-arrive boss.
- Still very early Monday, accompany the two supervisors to the department and help them advise the staff of the change. If possible, assure the employees that their jobs remain as secure as always.

- Stress that a true "open door" will be maintained, especially during this difficult week.
- Answer any reasonable (and nonconfidential) questions that the staff may have.
- Visit the department regularly throughout the week to remain visible to the staff and deal with their concerns.
- On the following Monday, personally introduce the new manager to the business office staff.

Chapter 5

Cases in Health Care Supervision

GROUP 1

Primary Focus: PEOPLE
Secondary Focus: TASK

P/T-01-01

Topic Emphasis: Change Management
Additional Topics: Communication, Leadership,
Motivation

Here We Go Again

The position of business office manager at Memorial Hospital has been a "hot seat," changing incumbents frequently. When the position was vacated last May, the four most senior employees in the department were interviewed. All were told that since they were at the top of grade and the compensation structure for new supervisors had "not yet caught up with that of other jobs," the position would not involve an increase in pay. All four refused the position, and all were given the impression that they were not really considered fully qualified anyway, but that they might be considered for supervision again at a later date.

That same month a new business office manager was hired from the outside, and the four senior employees were instructed to "show the new boss all they know." Over the following several months, the finance director told all four employees that they had "come along very well" and would be considered for the manager's position should it come open again.

In October of that same year the manager resigned. However, none of the four senior employees got the job; the process described above was repeated, and again a new manager was hired from the outside.

Questions

1. How do you believe the four senior employees would feel, having gone through the foregoing process twice?
2. What do you believe would be the attitudes of the business office staff toward the organization?
3. What do you believe would be the attitudes of the four senior employees toward the finance director?
4. Is the apparent inequity in the organization's wage and salary structure at all justifiable? Why, or why not?

P/T-01-02

Topic Emphasis: Change Management
Additional Topics: Communication, Leadership, Supervisory Authority

---

Boss? Who Needs One?

Kay Morgan is assigned to the reception desk at Community Hospital. Her job also includes sorting incoming mail for distribution, and metering and bundling all outgoing mail. She has been doing this same job since the hospital opened nearly 15 years ago. She always worked independently and was never assigned to any particular supervisor. She never appeared on an organization chart, and she considered the administrator, whom she rarely saw, to be her only "boss."

During a period of internal growth it was considered necessary to establish the position of business manager. You are hired from the outside to fill this new position. One of the activities placed under your direct supervision is Morgan's mail and reception area.

You cannot tell from your initial visit with Morgan if her seemingly quiet and stern manner is natural to her or perhaps indicates resentment. Your visit was not preceded by any announcement concerning your arrival as her supervisor.

Instructions

Develop an approach that will help you "start out on the right foot" with Kay Morgan. Do not assume at the outset that she *will* resist your authority. You actually have no idea of how she will react, although your showing up without notice does create some basis for concern on her part.

P/T - 01 - 03

Topic Emphasis: Change Management
Additional Topics: Communication, Meetings,
Supervisory Authority

It Wasn't *My* Decision

Within the finance division of City Hospital a problem developed in the processing of receiving reports from the receipt of incoming material to the completion of payment. The purchasing manager, Mr. Sampson, first recognized the problem and pointed it out to the assistant administrator. Sampson said he believed he understood the situation and knew how it should be corrected. However, five different departments were involved.

The assistant administrator directed Sampson to "get together with the other four supervisors and work out a solution."

On extremely short notice Sampson called a meeting of the affected supervisors. Only two of the four were able to attend; the others were out of the building when Sampson decided to get together. Nevertheless the three persons who were present went to work on the problem.

The three supervisors developed a solution which required no implementation on their part but called upon the other two supervisors to take all of the required action. Sampson put the results of their decision in a memo directed to the two supervisors who were expected to translate the decision into action.

Questions

1. Assuming the solution Sampson and his companions arrived at was the most reasonable answer available, could there be any legitimate reasons for resistance from the two supervisors who were expected to carry it out?
2. If you were one of the two supervisors left out of the decision process, how would you react to the "directive" from Sampson? What would you do about it?

P/T-01-04

Topic Emphasis: Change Management
Additional Topics: Communication, Leadership, Motivation

The Promotion

With considerable advance notice, your hospital's director of medical records resigned to take a similar position in a hospital in another state. Within the department it was assumed that you, the assistant director, would be appointed director. However, a month after your boss's departure the department was still running without a director. Day-to-day operations apparently had been left in your hands ("apparently," because nothing had been said to you), but the hospital's assistant administrator had begun to make some of the administrative decisions affecting medical records.

After another month had passed you learned "through the grapevine" that the hospital had interviewed several candidates for the position of director of medical records. Nobody had been hired, however.

During the next several weeks you tried several times to discuss your uncertain status with the assistant administrator. Each time you tried you were put off; once you were told simply to "keep doing what you're now doing."

Four months after the director's departure you were promoted to director of medical records. The first instruction you received from the assistant administrator was to abolish the position of assistant director.

Questions

1. Would your employees' view of you when you were finally promoted likely be the same as it would have been had you been promoted immediately? Why, or why not?
2. What effects, if any, could the delay have on your ability to fill the position of director effectively?

P/T-02-01

Topic Emphasis:	Communication
Additional Topics:	Change Management, Meetings, Motivation

Noisy Alone, Quiet Together

As the admitting supervisor newly hired from outside the hospital, it did not take you long to discover that morale in the department had been at a low ebb for quite some time. As you undertook to become acquainted with your employees by meeting with each of them one by one, you quickly became inundated with complaints and other evidences of discontent. Most of the complaints concerned problems with administration, the business office, and the loose admitting practices of physicians, but there were also a few complaints by admitting staff about other members of the department and a couple of thinly veiled charges concerning admitting personnel who "carry tales to administration."

In listening to the problems it occurred to you that there were a number of common threads running through them, and that a great deal of misunderstanding could be cleared up if the gripes were aired in open fashion with the entire group. You then planned a staff meeting for that purpose and asked all employees to be prepared to air their complaints—except those involving specific other staff members—at the meeting. Most of your employees seemed to think such a staff meeting was a good idea, and several assured you they would be ready to speak up.

Your first staff meeting, however, turned out to be brief. When offered the opportunity to air their gripes, nobody spoke.

The results—silence—were the same at your next staff meeting four weeks later, although in the intervening period you were steadily bombarded with complaints from individuals. This experience left you frustrated because you regarded many of the complaints as problems of the group rather than problems of individuals.

Questions

1. What can you do to get the group off dead center and to open up about what is bothering them?
2. How might you approach the specific problem of one or more of your employees carrying complaints outside of the department, that is, "carrying tales to administration"?

P/T-02-02

Topic Emphasis:	Communication
Additional Topics:	Delegation, General Management Practice, Supervisory Authority

---

The Orphan Supplies

When Jerry Bennett joined the John James Memorial Hospital staff as an administrative intern he was assigned to study the organization's structure and the apportionment of departmental responsibilities.

Early in his travels about the hospital to visit the supervisors of various departments, Jerry encountered a condition that disturbed him. In the basement of the main building, just outside of central supply, several dozen large cartons of paper products were stored in the corridor. The large cartons were stacked three deep against the wall along nearly 200 feet of the corridor. Although the corridor was wider than most and the cartons did not impede normal traffic, materials stored there placed the hospital in violation of local fire codes.

Because examining departmental responsibilities was part of his basic charge, Jerry decided to see if he could determine who was responsible for this material and find out why it could not be stored elsewhere. Since the supplies were stored outside of central supply, he made that department his first stop.

The manager of central supply explained, rather indignantly, that the boxes belonged to purchasing and stores; they had put them there because there was no room in their own storeroom. Since the boxes had been undisturbed for some months, it was probably a case of "purchasing fouling up and over-ordering again."

Jerry next visited purchasing where he asked the manager about the supplies. His answer: "Those belong to central supply. They did not know what to do with them, so they just stuck them in the hall as usual."

Jerry Bennett's investigation hit a dead end when he could find no paperwork that could tell him to which department the supplies belonged. The purchase order and accounting's record of payment were both on file. However, the purchase requisition had been only partially completed; there were no signatures on it, and the receiving copy of the purchase order was nowhere to be found.

What Jerry found most disturbing was that of the four products that made up this cache of material, one of them represented a ten-year supply of the item.

Questions

1. What likely systems problems has Jerry begun to uncover?
2. What can be said about the state of departmental authority-versus-responsibility in the case of the supplies?

P/T-02-03

Topic Emphasis:	Communication
Additional Topics:	Leadership, Motivation, People Problems

The Silencer

James Argus, a management consultant, was engaged by the board of directors of a small rural hospital to study communication within the organization and to assess employee attitude. He was to focus especially on the attitudes of supervisors and managers.

Argus arranged to hold informal discussion meetings, essentially "rap sessions," with the entire management group each Monday. So as not to disrupt operations more than necessary it was arranged for Argus to meet with half of the management group from 8:30 to 10:00 A.M. and the other half from 10:30 until noon. He was to do this each week for several weeks, while visiting the facility on other occasions to study organization structure and various aspects of departmental activity. The administrator told Argus in advance that he doubted the sessions would accomplish much; his management group consisted mostly of "close-mouthed people" who opened up only with great difficulty. Thus forewarned, Argus launched his first Monday session with some discussion-oriented case material which he hoped would get people talking.

After the first two Mondays Argus felt he may as well have been in the room alone. Each group was as silent as the other. The only comments made were strictly related to the case material he had brought along.

On the first two Mondays the administrator attended the earlier session, as did a dozen or more other people of varying management levels, including the hospital's second-in-command who served in the dual capacity of assistant administrator and personnel director.

However, the administrator was absent from the third early session, and Argus finally managed to create an opening in the wall that had confronted him. Evidently encouraged by something brought up in a case discussion, one supervisor began to relate a problem based on an incident that had apparently left him in a bad light in his employees' eyes and had caused embarrassment for two other supervisors. Although the supervisor mentioned no names, the story's disguise was sufficiently thin for the several participants—and their errors—to be recognizable. The discussion, however, was rational, if somewhat spirited, and a number of people made favorable comments to Argus after the session was over.

The people in the late morning session also opened up, fully as enthusiastically as those in the earlier group. Argus could only guess that a few comments had been exchanged between sessions.

When Argus arrived for the fourth Monday's sessions he was greeted by dead silence and long faces. There were several latecomers, and he noted several absences. The assistant administrator was there, but the administrator was absent. The late morning group was fully as silent as the earlier group, and there was one change in this group—the administrator was now a participant.

For the rest of the series of sessions the assistant administrator stayed with the early group, and the administrator remained with the later group. After the seventh scheduled session Argus called a halt to the series. Four straight sessions had produced little more than silence, which, along with facial expressions and other body language, told him a great deal about the organization.

Questions

1. What do you think may have caused both groups to revert to silence after "opening up" in the third session?
2. What might Argus have been able to infer from the behavior of the two discussion groups?

P/T-02-04

> *Topic Emphasis:* Communication
> *Additional Topics:* Leadership, Personal Effectiveness, Supervisory Authority

---

Get Back with You in a Minute

You are the laundry manager at Community Hospital and you report to the director of support services. You have just been through a particularly trying week, and you have concluded that your relationship with the director of support services is not in the best of shape. To review the contacts you had, or tried to have, with your boss in the past week:

- Monday morning a personnel problem arose which you figured was going to require severe disciplinary action. You thought you should clear it with your boss. However, you could not reach him. You called his office three times; each time you spoke with his secretary who said she would leave word for him to return your call. Monday ended without response from the boss.
- On Tuesday you encountered your boss in a basement corridor when he was going in the opposite direction. You told him you needed to

see him on a matter of some importance, and you moved directly toward him, nearly blocking his passage. Without slowing, he detoured around you and called back over his shoulder, "Something's up—can't stop. Get back with you in a minute." You did not see him again that day. When you called his office you were told he was in a meeting.

- On Wednesday morning you decided to visit the boss's office. However, you found that he had two visitors. He saw you at the door and shrugged, smiled faintly, and waved you away.
- On Wednesday afternoon you telephoned the boss's office. His secretary must have been away from her desk because he answered his own phone and immediately told you he was tied up with someone. He said he would "—buzz you back as soon as I'm free." You remained nearly an hour after quitting time but he did not "buzz you back." When you left you noticed that his office was dark.
- On Thursday you made no effort to contact the director of support services. Rather, since the item you had been holding open since Monday morning was still plaguing you and someone needed an answer, you went ahead and took care of it using your best judgment. You felt that you might be overstepping your authority, but you knew that continuing to delay a decision would only cause harm.
- On Friday you encountered the director twice while you were moving about the lower level of the hospital. The first time you told him you needed to get a few minutes of his time. He told you he was on his way to the administrator's office, but he would get back with you shortly. Nothing. On the second occasion he saw you before you saw him, and he called out, "Hey, we need to get together for a little bit. I'm on my way to an administrative staff meeting, but catch me in my office at about 4:00." However, the boss was not in his office at 4:00 P.M. Neither was he there at 4:30, the normal quitting time, nor was he there at 5:00 P.M. when you left for the weekend. You learned on the way out of the building that the administrative staff meeting had ended at 3:30.

Upon review you felt that the week, taken in its entirety, looked pretty grim. Unfortunately, you have experienced too many such weeks.

Instructions

There are two general approaches you can adopt to the problem of working for the director of support services. You can:

a. mount an all-out effort to "get his attention," concentrating on getting him into situations in which he cannot avoid dealing with you for at least a few minutes; or

b. decide to "do your own thing," doing your job as you see fit and handling all decisions that arise regardless of where they fall relative to your scope of authority.

Determine how you might go about developing both of these approaches, including what specific steps you might consider in either or both cases, and identifying all possible pitfalls and hazards present in both.

P/T-02-05

Topic Emphasis: Communication
Additional Topics: Meetings, People Problems, Supervisory Authority

---

Your Word Against His

You are at a meeting which your department head is chairing. Also present are another department head and four other supervisors. The subject of the meeting is the manner in which the institution's supervisors are to conduct themselves during the present union-organizing campaign.

Your department head makes a statement concerning one way in which supervisors should conduct themselves. You are surprised to hear his statement because earlier that day you read a legal opinion which described this particular action as probably illegal.

You interrupt your department head with, "Pardon me, but I don't believe it can really be done quite that way. I'm certain it would leave us open to an unfair labor practice charge."

Obviously irritated at being interrupted, your department head says sharply, "This isn't open to discussion. You're wrong."

You open your mouth to speak again, but you are cut short by an angry glance.

You are absolutely certain that your boss is wrong; he had inadvertently turned around a couple of words and described a "cannot-do" as a "can-do." Unfortunately you are in a conference room full of people, and the document which could prove your point is in your office.

Question

What can you do to set the matter straight without prejudicing yourself with your department head?

P/T-02-06 (E)

Topic Emphasis: Communication
Additional Topics: Motivation, People Problems

Is There Any Truth in This Matter of . . .?

This is a group exercise, best suited to groups of 15 or more persons. The instructions are intended for the instructor or group coordinator. The exercise itself, similar to a common party game, is intended to illustrate what happens to a story or a bit of information when it is passed from person to person.

First you will need some small slips of paper, one for each person who will participate in the exercise. On three slips of paper write the word *starter,* and on one of these slips draw a circle around that word. On one-fourth to one-third of the remaining slips of paper write the word *stopper.* On all other slips of paper write the word *spreader.* Fold all slips of paper so the words cannot be seen and mix them in a box, or simply scatter the slips face down on a tabletop.

Tell the group you are going to give them a 15-minute break; this exercise seems to work best if it does in fact take place during an actual break from class. Tell them that they are being asked to participate in a rumor-spreading exercise. When the break begins they should each draw a slip of paper and respond as follows:

a. The three *starters* are to come to you immediately for instructions.
b. The few *stoppers* should carry no tales regardless of what they hear. They will undoubtedly participate in a certain amount of social conversation during the break, but anything they hear concerning activities afoot in the organization should not be repeated. They are to

serve as rumor stoppers, assuring that what they hear does not go beyond them.

c. Those identified as *spreaders* should repeat any organizationally related tales they hear during the break. Each spreader should pass along the story at least twice, that is, tell the tale twice whether to individuals or to small groups, and preferably more often if time permits.

When the three *starters* join you for instructions, let them know that you are using the person who drew the circled word as the true *starter*. Explain to the three people that the function of two of them is to prevent the rest of the group from knowing who the true *starter* of the exercise really is. While the four of you are together, give the true *starter* exactly two minutes to read and absorb the following:

The Story

The administrator had a visitor this morning. Hard-looking man, businesslike from the word go. He's never been here before, but I think I remember seeing him over at County General when I worked there.

He's some kind of consultant or efficiency expert or something, and if we're in for it like they were at County—watch out. Back at County this guy and some others showed up and after a while—wow, you wouldn't believe the heads that rolled and the mess they made with their computers.

He and the administrator sure spent a long time in the business office. I heard them say something about billings—I think this guy is some kind of an accountant, too. There've been a lot of things said lately about sky-high costs in accounting; you can bet we're going to see machinery coming in and people going out.

After the *starter* has two minutes to absorb the story, retrieve the written version and let the three people join the others on break. The two false *starters* are to assume the role of *spreader* during the exercise. The *starter* should be asked to tell the story at least three times.

Allow at least 15 minutes for the exercise from the time the *starter* joins the group.

Afterward

Open the exercise for group discussion. By either requesting volunteers or asking specific people, bring out into the open as many variations of the story as can be identified. After doing this, read to the group the text of the story as it was seen by the *starter*. During subsequent discussion, ask the group to consider the implications of the following questions:

1. What probably causes a story to become distorted as it passes from person to person?
2. What kinds of information seem to experience the most distortion as such a story is passed around?
3. What should you do if such a story—but a *real* one—reaches your ears?
4. Having gone through this exercise, what is your assessment of the value of the organization's "grapevine" or "rumor mill"?

P/T-02-07

Topic Emphasis:	Communication
Additional Topics:	Motivation, People Problems, Supervisory Authority

---

Aren't You Happy Here?

Helen Bowen was head nurse on days in the hospital's largest medical/surgical unit. She reported directly to Lydia Clark, who reported in turn to Mary Lyons, the director of nursing service. This three-level relationship had existed for five years. The director maintained constant contact with the lower levels of management on the day shift, but on the evening and night shifts her close contacts did not extend below the level of supervisor.

An opportunity came to Lydia Clark when she was offered the position of director of inservice education. She accepted immediately. Although this was but a lateral move, it meant the fulfillment of a long-held ambition. She was to be replaced by Jane Miller who had been evening supervisor for two years.

Lydia Clark had been aware for some time that Helen Bowen was discontented with a number of things in nursing service. Helen and Lydia got along well, to the point where Helen had at times suggested that if she were ever to lose Lydia as an immediate supervisor she might start looking for another position. Lydia did not want to see Helen leave because she considered her a capable employee, but neither did she wish to lose out on the inservice education position simply because one employee preferred her over other supervisors.

Lydia wanted to maintain the stability of the day shift and make the transfer of supervision as smooth as possible. In a series of personal contacts she advised Jane Miller completely about the activities of the unit. Upon mention of Helen Bowen, Lydia said that this particular head nurse, who was capable and a definite asset to the department, may be considering looking for another job.

Shortly after assuming the position of day supervisor, Jane Miller told Mary Lyons she had reliable information that Helen Bowen was actively seeking another position. Almost at once the director sent a brief note to Helen wanting to know if it was true that she was thinking of leaving and asking her what the trouble was.

Accusations and hard feelings followed. When tempers began to clear, each party was able to state her position as follows:

Helen Bowen: Sure, I've been discontented with a few things, but as long as my immediate supervisor knows I feel this way that's as far as it should go. I feel uneasy having the director know I'm thinking of possibly leaving.

Lydia Clark: Mrs. Miller was stepping into my position. I felt she had the right to know that one of her key people was probably unhappy.

Jane Miller: I feel the director has the right to know that one of our head nurses might leave.

Mary Lyons: If one of our head nurses is unhappy on the job to the point of thinking about leaving, I believe I should try to do something about it.

Questions

1. Assume that Lydia knew of Helen's discontent for some time and that she has managed to work with her and forestall her departure. Examine the related interpersonal transactions that took place after the reorganization: Clark to Miller; Miller to Lyons; Lyons to Bowen. Were any or all of these transactions justified?

2. Should each of these transactions have been governed by *the right to confidence* or by *the need to know?* Why?

P/T-03-01

      Topic Emphasis: Criticism and Discipline
  Additional Topics: Communication, Delegation, People
                           Problems

You're It

The small combination intensive care and coronary care unit usually contained at least one patient, but rarely were there more than three patients in the four-bed unit. Consequently, on most days the unit was staffed with a single registered nurse. On the night shift this assignment fell to Theresa Ross.

Ross made it plain from the moment she was assigned that she did not want to work in the unit. The reason, she contended, was that she did not work well under conditions of stress and tension. She felt she was a capable general-duty nurse, but she claimed she knew herself well enough to realize that she became disoriented under pressure. She did not want to be put in a position in which she might make the wrong decision at a crucial time. She took her argument to the night supervisor who listened but said she could do nothing about it since Theresa was the only RN on nights who had completed the coronary care training program. Ross then took her argument to the director of nursing from whom she received the same response.

One night when there were three patients in the unit, two of whom had just been admitted that night, one patient died under questionable circumstances. A coronary patient, the man had been admitted by a surgeon who had simply been the first physician available. There was some question as to the appropriateness of the surgeon's orders, and the man had died before a cardiologist could be reached. However, there was no question about the misinterpretation of the physician's orders and the almost total misapplication of his instructions.

The following day the director of nursing conducted a cursory investigation which included conversations with Ross, the night supervisor, and the physician on the case. Then, with administration's concurrence, Theresa Ross was fired. She was told that the records indicated extremely poor case management on her part and that the hospital could not afford the risk of a repetition of such an occurrence.

Instructions

Comment on all aspects of the case. Be sure to include consideration of the following:

● how "right" or "wrong" you consider each involved person to be relative to the outcome;
● how Theresa Ross might possibly have protected herself from dismissal;
● whether you believe personal characteristics such as Ross's acknowledged weakness under pressure are valid to consider when assigning people, or if "a nurse is a nurse and should be expected to function wherever she is assigned, as long as she has had the proper training."

P/T-03-02 (R)

Topic Emphasis: Criticism and Discipline
Additional Topics: Communication, Hiring, Rules and Policies

The Case of Joan H.

Joan H. was a technician in the laboratory of City Hospital. Her immediate supervisor was George P., a supervising technician who looked after the duties of the blood-collecting team and also worked as a member of that team. George reported to Gloria W., unit manager of the laboratory.

Joan had worked at City Hospital for five months when she was discharged for chronic tardiness. The unit manager initiated the firing, and the supervising technician concurred. When the matter was turned over to personnel it was pointed out that on three prior occasions Joan was given written warnings for punching in more than 30 minutes late. Gloria also suggested there were numerous other occurrences that had been overlooked or had resulted in verbal warnings only.

Joan complained to personnel and administration that the starting time for the blood-collecting team was too early for her (the team began at 6:30 A.M.). As a divorcee, she said, she had the responsibility of looking after one child, and even though she lived with relatives she had difficulty getting out in time to get to the hospital by 6:30 A.M. She further stated that when she was hired George had led her to believe the job on the blood-collecting team was temporary, and there would be an opening for her in the lab itself in two or three months. It would make a considerable difference, she said, starting work at 8:00 A.M.

Gloria had criticized George for being too lenient and stepping outside of hospital policy. On the occasion of the first tardiness he delivered the required oral warning; however, on the second and third instances he repeated the oral warning but did not issue written warnings. It was only on the prompting of Gloria, who insisted that policy be followed in all matters, that George began to document warnings for tardiness.

According to policy, the fourth written warning for tardiness constituted grounds for dismissal. On review of each written warning Joan was so advised. Following the fourth warning Joan was fired.

Although Gloria and George both admitted the likely mention of a regular technician job, they were both convinced there had been no promises to that effect. This contention was supported by the employment manager who had also discussed with Joan the possibility of stepping into a different job should one become available.

Joan took her complaint to the state and claimed that her firing was unwarranted and unfair. Although she had been late a few times, she said, she usually worked late an equal amount of time and never failed to do her assigned tasks. (Discussions with George cast some doubt on this statement. George claimed that on days when Joan was not there at 6:30 A.M., he and another technician had to cover more territory to make up for the missing Joan.)

Joan also charged that the written policy meant very little; she had been late several times early in her employment, and these did not result in written warnings. She charged management in general and Gloria in particular with using the policy as an excuse to get rid of her.

Instructions

This activity involves four roles. These may be assumed by individuals or by groups (with each group ideally channeling its comments through a spokesperson). The role positions are:

1. *Joan*—You believe you were unjustly dismissed, that you were treated with prejudice, especially by Gloria, and you are asking to be reinstated.
2. *Gloria*—You believe Joan was discharged for cause, that she was treated as any other employee, and that the dismissal should stand.

3. *George*—You see yourself as a supervisor who cares about people and always extends the benefit of the doubt. You also believe, however, that Joan was given every chance to correct her behavior and that she should not be reinstated.
4. *The State Employment Commission Hearing Examiner*—You are to question Joan, Gloria, and George to whatever extent you believe necessary and recommend that Joan's dismissal be either sustained or overturned. You must state the reasons for your decision.

P/T-03-03

Topic Emphasis: Criticism and Discipline
Additional Topics: Communication, Labor Relations, Rules and Policies

---

Dismissal for Cause

William Short is administrator for Benton Memorial Hospital, a 120-bed institution and one of two hospitals in a small city. He has been there for eight months. Prior to his arrival the hospital ran for four months without an administrator following the former administrator's abrupt and unexplained departure.

The last administrator appeared to have been extremely well liked by his management group; at the same time he was at constant odds with his board of directors. The former administrator was considered easygoing, low-key in style, and slow to act in many matters.

William Short stands in direct contrast; his pace is rapid, and his manner is brusque and forceful. It is generally believed that Short was brought into the organization to apply pressure to the management team and perhaps weed out certain individuals. Therefore, Short was greeted with some apprehension and resentment, and his personal style has done nothing to help reverse those early impressions.

Among several members of supervision who remained cool toward Short was Clara Jackson. Jackson was with the hospital some nine years and for the last five years was emergency room supervisor.

It took William Short the better part of eight months to work his lengthy priority list down to one particular problem: overtime authorization and approval. One of the departments with consistent overtime use out of proportion to the rest of the hospital was the emergency room.

Short asked Jackson to turn over her overtime logs. These included the names of the persons authorized to work overtime, dates, hours, and authorizing initials of either the director or the assistant director of nursing. Mrs. Jackson's cool response was that she had misplaced the logs, and that she saw no reason why he should have to have them anyway.

All he had to do, she claimed, was check the time cards through the payroll department. Nevertheless, Short repeated his request several times and finally directed Jackson to stop stalling and locate the logs.

When Short received the overtime logs he was first struck by the fact that all the entries were in the same color ink and the same style of writing. This suggested they may have all been entered at once. This suggestion became a near certainty when he noticed that the date on which the most recent log pages were started was some three weeks before the date appearing in the lower left corner as the reprinting date of the form. Further investigation revealed that the initials of the director and the assistant director of nursing service were not authentic.

When Short confronted Jackson she first denied creating the logs and then reversed her story and admitted doing so. She claimed she did so because Short was applying pressure, and she was afraid to admit she lost the originals. She resisted Short's allegation that she had never maintained the logs in the first place but had simply authorized overtime herself, entered it on the time cards, and put it through without following policy.

Short's allegations were largely supported by the director and the assistant director of nursing service who claimed it had been a year or more since they were last asked to authorize overtime for the emergency room. When asked why this did not seem to bother them, their answer suggested that under the last administrator policies such as the one for overtime authorization were neither observed nor enforced.

On the basis of violation of hospital policy and falsification of records, Short discharged Jackson. Jackson strongly objected to the firing and appealed to several board members through common acquaintances. Her personal appeals were unsuccessful, so she filed a complaint with the State Employment Commission charging the firing was arbitrary and unfair.

William Short was called before a State Employment Commission hearing to show cause why Clara Jackson should not be reinstated.

Instructions

Consider all the information in the case and render a decision which either:

a. supports the firing of Jackson, or
b. reinstates Jackson.

Explain why you made your decision and on what you base the decision. Also, identify the management errors which permitted the situation to occur.

P/T-03-04

Topic Emphasis: Criticism and Discipline
Additional Topics: Communication, Meetings, Motivation

When Do You Stop Being General?

You are supervisor of central transcription at City General Hospital. Your group includes several transcriptionists who handle all the dictation from the laboratory and x-ray and the typing for several department managers as well as all medical record transcription.

You are in the habit of holding a brief informational meeting with your staff early each month. At your June meeting you felt obligated to point out that quality was slipping and typing errors were on the increase, and that more care had to be taken with typing. At your July meeting you made the following statement: "The overall quality of typing has not improved at all in the last month; in fact, it has gotten worse. I expect all of you to begin improving your typing quality immediately."

It is now almost time for your August meeting. In your estimation, typing quality has not improved in the least.

Questions

1. Do you continue to deal with the group at large? Why, or why not?
2. How do you believe you might approach the problem of making your criticism increasingly more specific?

P/T-03-05

Topic Emphasis: Criticism and Discipline
Additional Topics: Communication, Motivation, People Problems

---

The Dodger

Jane Wilson had considerable difficulty developing the schedule for her nursing unit for the coming two weeks. The nursing department was in a marginal position overall as far as available nurses were concerned, so her flexibility was limited. To make matters worse, within hours after Jane issued the newest schedule Alice Johnson, a part-time licensed practical nurse, submitted a request for a personal day on one of the days she was scheduled to work.

The request caused Jane to realize she had been seeing Alice's name in connection with schedule difficulties often in recent months. Looking back over the preceding six months' schedules she discovered that the current request was the fifth time in six months that Alice had requested time off on a scheduled weekend day. Even more significant was the pattern of Alice's use of sick time. She had called in sick four times, all of these on Saturdays or Sundays. All in all Alice had worked only about half of the weekend days she was scheduled to work over a period of six months.

Jane was displeased with Alice's attendance and unhappy with herself for not discovering the problem sooner. She felt she had to talk with Alice about it, but she also felt that her unit could ill afford to lose a nurse. Nevertheless she believed that she could not allow Alice's attendance pattern to continue uncorrected.

Questions

1. What are the hazards Jane faces in:
   a. dealing firmly with Alice's behavior?
   b. ignoring Alice's absences and saying nothing?
2. Assuming Jane is seriously considering talking with Alice, how might she approach the subject of the attendance problem?

P/T-03-06

Topic Emphasis: Criticism and Discipline
Additional Topics: Communication, Leadership, People Problems

An Act of Negligence

This morning you entered the workroom of your nursing unit just in time to see Jenny Walters, an aide whom you considered a usually careful worker, commit an act of negligence. There was little room for doubt, and Jenny's behavior resulted in several pieces of costly glassware being broken before your eyes.

In addition to Jenny, three more of your employees were present when you entered and witnessed the incident.

Questions

1. Should you:
   a. reprimand Jenny on the spot, while the incident is fresh and the other employees can take your criticism as a warning?
   b. separate Jenny from the group and deliver the reprimand in private?
2. Which option did you choose? Why?
3. How can you improve upon your chosen option?

P/T-05-01 (R)

Topic Emphasis: Delegation
Additional Topics: Change Management, Communication,
Supervisory Authority

A Case of Management Prerogative

Mary Alexander has a good work record as a staff nurse in medical/surgical unit 3-A. She has been with the hospital several years. Apparently she is satisfied with her assignment, and she seems to enjoy what she does. She is happy with her salary increases and feels that she has been treated fairly in relation to other employees.

Last Monday, with less than one day's notice, Mary was permanently transferred to pediatrics. The transfer was made without explanation; there was no attempt by the head nurse or the day supervisor to find out if Mary would object to the transfer. Her classification and salary are to remain unchanged. The job in pediatrics is as important as the one in medical/surgical, but she was not consulted about the transfer.

Mary sought out the supervisor and asked why she was transferred. She was told that her skills were needed in pediatrics and that she must go where the needs are the greatest. Mary objected, insisting that she had a right to be consulted about her assignment. The supervisor disagreed, saying that Mary should be prepared to work wherever placed at the convenience of the institution.

Instructions

The persons or groups assigned the roles of Mary and the day supervisor should pursue their arguments along the following lines:

Mary—Within reason, all employees should have something to say about where they are assigned.
Supervisor—All employees are paid to be of service to the patients as determined by the management of the institution and should be prepared to work where they are placed.

P/T-05-02

Topic Emphasis: Delegation
Additional Topics: Communication, Leadership

Given and Taken Away

You are manager of the business office at Unity Memorial Hospital. On Monday of this week your immediate supervisor, the assistant controller, assigned you to the task of coming up with a new technique for scheduling the several part-time people who handle registration and billing for the hospital's numerous clinics and outpatient activities. The essence of the assignment was:

I want you to come up with a new way of scheduling all of our part-timers. Make it a cyclic scheduling technique so we can repeat it over and over again in cycles of, say, 90 days. I want it so everyone has to take a fair share of the odd hours—the early shifts, the late clinics, and so on. I'd like to have the whole thing, including the first firm 90-day schedule, before the first of the month, but I'll take it whenever you can get it ready.

Three days passed before you were able to get seriously involved in the scheduling project, but things settled down and you discovered you were able to spend most of Thursday on the task. By late Thursday afternoon you felt that you had a workable process and a sample schedule fairly well outlined, but you thought you would like to clear up a couple of points with some of the people who would actually have to work to the schedule. You took a few minutes to visit a clerk on one of the afternoon clinics. The clerk frowned upon seeing your schedule and asked, "What are you guys trying to do, anyway?"

When asked what was meant by that remark, the clerk produced a schedule she had received just that morning. It bore the previous day's date and the assistant controller's initials in the lower right-hand corner. It looked like a cyclic schedule, but the cycle was 30 days rather than 90 days, and it did not call for the odd hours to be shared equally by all.

You obtained a copy of the schedule and went to see the assistant controller. He freely admitted that it was his work.

"But you asked me to do this," you said. "I've already spent several hours on it."

Your boss responded, "I know you did, but I had a little time on my hands and a couple of ideas came to me, so I went ahead and took care of it."

This was the third time in as many months that your immediate supervisor gave you a job with an indefinite deadline and then, without informing you, went ahead and did it himself in a manner different from his instructions to you.

Question

What can you do about the manner in which your boss "delegates" to minimize the chances of finding yourself in the same situation in the future?

P/T-05-03

Topic Emphasis: Delegation
Additional Topics: Communication, Motivation, People Problems

Where Are They When I Need Them?

Jenny Lee is head nurse on 3-west, a 40-bed geriatric unit which is nearly always fully occupied. Many of the patients spend several hours each day in wheelchairs, but most return to their beds for two or three hours in the afternoon.

Jenny has been concerned that her limited staff is only marginally able to fulfill all the needs of the elderly patients. She has spoken with many patients concerning needs that volunteers could possibly fill for them, and she has developed a list of volunteers who indicated they could make themselves available to help. Jenny developed a 30-day schedule for volunteer support.

On the first day of the schedule three of the five volunteers did not show up. On the second day, two did not appear. Only one showed up on each of the third and fourth days, and on the fifth day there were no volunteers present in the unit. Jenny abandoned her schedule.

Jenny was thoroughly discouraged by the volunteers' lack of dependability. Further, since Jenny made no secret of her volunteer program, a number of patients were similarly discouraged, and several complained.

Questions

1. What has Jenny been doing wrong?
2. What might she consider doing to correct the situation that she has gotten herself into?

P/T-05-04

Topic Emphasis: Delegation
Additional Topics: Communication, Motivation,
Supervisory Authority

The Unnecessary Task

The medical record department of Memorial Hospital was considered able to function for a day or two at a time without a supervisor when necessary. However, when Mrs. James, the manager of medical records, was hospitalized for several weeks administration asked Guy Smith, the director of admissions, to look in on medical records on a regular basis. (In his previous position in a smaller hospital Smith had supervised both admitting and medical records.)

About noon one day Smith noticed a completed form entitled "Daily Census Report" on the corner of the desk of a clerk in the medical records department. It caught his eye because in his months at the hospital the only census report he had seen was the computer-generated report he received each morning. He became even more curious when he noticed that the hand-generated report bore this day's date. He asked the clerk who created the report and why.

"I do it," she said, "but I don't really know why." She proceeded to describe the process: Each morning she took the previous day's record department count of admissions and discharges and merged it with information obtained from copies of the midnight census report generated by the head nurse in each nursing unit. This took her about an hour and a half each day.

Smith asked, "Who uses this report?"

"I don't think anybody uses it."

"Then let me put it this way," said Smith, his frustration beginning to show, "who receives the report?"

"Nobody," the clerk answered. She went on to explain that some time earlier the hospital experienced problems with its data processing system and certain census information was being lost. Her then-supervisor, Mrs. Victor, showed her how to do the report and told her where to leave it. For about four weeks the report was picked up faithfully at noon every day.

"Why hasn't it been discontinued?" asked Smith.

"It *was* discontinued, once," the clerk answered. "By me. And I got into plenty of trouble over it. It got picked up regularly only for about four weeks. After that, before I knew it I had eight or nine of them on my desk. I tried to ask Mrs. Victor about it, but I couldn't get an answer—you couldn't get her to stand still for ten seconds—so I just stopped doing it on my own because I couldn't see any sense in it. Then about a week after I stopped someone came looking for it. When Mrs. Victor found out I dropped it she gave me the chewing out of my life and said that I'd better never do anything like that again without a direct order."

Smith said, "But Mrs. Victor has been gone for more than a year. Did you mention this to Mrs. James?"

"Yes, but I'm not sure it ever sank in. She's just as busy as Mrs. Victor ever was, and the only people who seem to be able to get her attention for more than a minute at a time are administration and the doctors. She said she'd look into it, but I haven't heard anything. And I'm not sticking my neck out again."

Guy Smith spent a few more minutes with the clerk looking over some of the reports. In that time he discovered that the clerk had done neat, accurate work, taking as long as 90 minutes a day, for nearly 25 months. And 23 months' worth of this work was never seen by anyone other than the clerk herself.

Questions

1. Who do you see as responsible for the perpetuation of the unnecessary task? Why?
2. What fundamental errors or shortcomings do you believe caused this to happen?
3. What should Smith do with his newly acquired information?

P/T-05-05

Topic Emphasis: Delegation
Additional Topics: Communication, Supervisory Authority

Assignment and Reassignment

Carol Ames was director of inservice education at James Memorial Hospital. She reported to Ann Baker, assistant director of nursing service, who in turn reported to the director of nursing, Helen Cary.

One morning as Carol sat working alone in her office, Helen Cary entered and said, "Come and have a cup of coffee, Carol. There's something I'd like to talk about with you."

After they got their coffee and found seats in a quiet corner of the cafeteria, the following conversation took place:

Cary—How busy are you these days, Carol? There's something I'd very much like you to do for me.
Ames—I'm rather loaded right now. I don't have a great deal of time to spare.

Cary—I didn't think your teaching schedule was too full right now, at least not since you completed the nursing leadership program. What's taking up your time?

Ames—It's true that my class schedule is only moderate right now. It was probably because of the slight dip in my workload that Ann just gave me a couple of new assignments.

Cary—Like what?

Ames—For one thing, she's given me just two weeks to compile a complete inventory of instructional materials and training aids throughout the hospital. Also, she's having me do a report concerning the costs of supplying hospital education programs to all employees. It has to be submitted to the State Hospital Association next month, and it's rather long and complicated.

Cary—Well, it has suddenly become very important—and I think perhaps you knew this was coming—that we get busy with the development of our new nursing audit criteria. We're coming under sudden pressure from administration to do something about audit, and we don't have a great deal of time in which to do it.

Ames—Where do I fit in?

Cary—Since you're in the best position to do so, I want you to take charge of the nursing audit committee. It will be up to you to convene the committee as necessary and get the criteria developed on time.

Ames—But what do I do about the other things? The inventory and the cost report? Surely I'm not going to have time for everything.

Cary—Of course you won't have time for everything. Ann will have to find some other way to get the cost report done, and the inventory will just have to wait.

Ames—Is Ann aware of all this?

Cary—No. I want you to tell her all about it. And please stress how important this audit committee activity really is.

At this point Cary excused herself. Carol got a second cup of coffee and pondered the situation. She felt that her immediate supervisor, Ann Baker, had been quite clear about what she wanted done over the coming weeks. However, Carol now found herself wondering how to convey to her boss that her assignment had been changed by a higher authority.

Questions

1. What fundamental management error was committed?
2. What do you believe Carol Ames should do (or try to do) about the situation which has been created?

P/T-07-01

Topic Emphasis: Hiring
Additional Topics: Communication, People Problems,
Rules and Policies

Choices

You have a position open in your department, and you have been presented with three candidates for consideration. All are equally qualified. They are:

1. A young woman, 19 years old, who has one child and is separated from her husband.
2. A woman, 31 years old, who has been unsuccessfully seeking work for several months and whose husband is disabled.
3. The daughter of a fellow employee. This young lady actually desires to get into a different department, but would like to have this job until there is an opening in the department of her choice.

Much of the little you know about the first two candidates (as noted above) is "forbidden information" in that you are not allowed to ask for it on an application or in an interview. However, the candidates themselves volunteered this information. What you know about the third person came to you from the fellow employee who wants you to hire her daughter.

Questions

1. What are the points of "forbidden information" referred to? Why are you not allowed to solicit this information?
2. What are some of the potential problems coming with the hiring of any of the three?
3. Under what circumstances would you likely rule out all three candidates?

P/T-07-02

Topic Emphasis: Hiring
Additional Topics: Communication, Rules and Policies,
Supervisory Authority

Shortage of Help

You are director of nursing service in a hospital which recently completed an expansion program and opened a new 36-bed medical/surgical unit. Recently you have not done too badly in keeping your nursing staff up to required levels in spite of a general shortage of nurses across the state, but the opening of the new unit has strained your resources to the extent where you are short several registered nurses. This shortage is particularly evident on the evening shift (3:00 P.M. to 11:00 P.M.); you have more than enough people willing to work days, and you have long had a thoroughly stable crew who prefer to work nights.

In response to your long-running recruiting efforts, a well-qualified registered nurse has applied for employment. You are impressed with her; she seems energetic and personable, and she is immediately available. Also, she is quite willing to take a position on the evening shift.

Unfortunately, while she is willing to work 3:00 P.M. to 11:00 P.M., she has also stated during her initial interview that she cannot agree to work any weekends. She will say only that weekend work causes severe inconvenience in her family life, and she repeats her willingness to work evenings, but only Monday through Friday.

You have not yet explained to her that scheduling practices in your hospital require everyone below the level of day, evening, or night supervisor to work every other weekend.

Questions

1. Conscious of your critical need for nursing help on evenings, what are you going to tell this applicant?
2. If you adhere to your scheduling policy and the nurse refuses the job, what problems will you be facing?

3. If you alter your scheduling policy and offer the applicant a Monday-through-Friday position which she accepts, what problems are you likely to face then?

P/T-08-01

Topic Emphasis: Labor Relations
Additional Topics: Decision Making, Rules and Policies, Supervisory Authority

---

Facts—or Opinion?

In the laboratory of the hospital, a group of unionized technicians normally performed numerous tests and distributed records of the results. Their supervisor, not a member of the union, usually did not do any routine work, but sometimes ran a few tests to check quality. This small amount of testing was understood to be part of his supervisory function.

When several employees arrived for work one day they saw that the supervisor had done some testing after hours. They thought that regular employees should have been offered overtime for this work. The contract provided for time-and-a-half for overtime, but did not guarantee any specific amount of overtime. The only reference to supervisors was the recognition clause which said they were not in the union; this did not specifically prohibit them from doing some work. As a matter of practice the hospital had never before permitted supervisors to do union work when no union employees were on the premises. The case went to arbitration, and the union argued:

- Although the contract said nothing specific about it, the recognition clause implied that supervisors could not do union work.
- In the past, when testing was required after regular hours, a union employee was asked to work overtime.

Administration replied:

- The work that the supervisor did came in after the employees had left, and it took him no more than 20 minutes. It would be unreasonable to recall an employee for so little work.

- Administration had successfully resisted the union's attempt to bar supervisors from doing such work during contract negotiations, which was why the contract said nothing about it.

Instructions

Imagine yourself in the position of an impartial arbitrator, and decide whether administration or the union is "right." Prepare to defend your decision with information from the case description.

P/T-08-02

Topic Emphasis: Labor Relations
Additional Topics: Communication, Decision Making, Leadership

---

The Forceful Organizer

You are the hospital's admitting supervisor. This morning you were called to attend a meeting concerned with possible union-organizing activity.

On your way to the meeting you observe a man (his back is to you, and you do not recognize him) backing one of the housekeepers into a corner. The man appears to be trying to get the housekeeper to take a card and a pen he is holding.

You cannot hear what is being said, but the housekeeper appears to be close to tears, and she is effectively trapped in the corner. Your first thought is of active solicitation of interest in a union election.

You move closer in an attempt to see the man's face.

Questions

1. What will you do if you recognize the man as an employee?
2. What will you do if you are certain that the man is *not* a hospital employee?
3. Whether or not you recognize the man as an employee, what should be your *first* action?

P/T-09-01

Topic Emphasis: Leadership
Additional Topics: Communication, Supervisory
Authority

The Bull of the Woods

As a supervisor in the maintenance department you report to the manager of building services.

The plate on the manager's desk saying "The Buck Stops Here" reasonably describes this person's approach to the job. He never avoids a decision or a problem, even of the most controversial or unpleasant sort, and for this you respect him.

However, the manager of building services makes his decisions in a vacuum with no input from any of his employees. He is apparently conscientious in his attempts to come up with the best solution each time, but when he transmits the instructions for carrying out his decisions he does so without giving you or anyone else the opportunity to provide the perspective of the person who has to translate the order into action.

Question

When you receive an order from "the bull of the woods" which you *know* is inappropriate—and assume you know so because you're much closer to the problem—how can you make yourself heard without deliberately rejecting his style of leadership?

P/T-13-01

Topic Emphasis: People Problems
Additional Topics: Change Management,
Communication, Decision Making

Linda's Dilemma

After having been a staff nurse for nearly five years, Linda James was given the position of nursing inservice education instructor. Linda and Carol Ross, the other inservice instructor, both reported to the hospital's director of staff development, Janice Carson.

It quickly became apparent to Linda that she was on her own as far as her orientation to the education position was concerned. Carson, a former professional educator responsible for education throughout the hospital, stayed away from areas requiring medical knowledge. The other instructor, Carol, was usually too busy to spend significant amounts of time with Linda. On the few occasions when Linda managed to isolate Carol for a few minutes' conversation, Carol's advice struck Linda as disorganized and, in some instances, inappropriate.

For her first several classroom appearances Linda functioned as assistant to Carol. After four such classes Linda found herself reluctantly concluding that her coinstructor had an inadequate grip on most essential teaching skills. Wondering if Carson had observed Carol's classroom manner, Linda asked some carefully framed questions of a number of frequent class attendees and learned that Carson never attended any of the classes put on by her instructors.

When she advanced to the point of doing classes on her own Linda began to discover that the greatest challenge she faced was correcting the misinformation dispensed by her fellow instructor in previous classes. Linda was alarmed; it seemed that Carol's approach to teaching was haphazard, misinformed, and consistently undermining that which had been taught correctly by others.

As she pondered her predicament Linda was forced to recognize two reasons why her observations would not be likely to register well with Carson:

a. Carol Ross and Janice Carson were close friends; in fact, Carson had been responsible for bringing Carol into the hospital.
b. As a professional educator coming from outside of health care, Carson had no basic medical orientation and was thus in no position to rule on the correctness of clinical information.

In short, the staff education department had no member of management who, with knowledge and without personal bias, could judge the appropriateness of any material presented by Carol Ross.

Questions

1. Short of stepping down and either leaving the hospital or returning to active nursing, how might Linda deal with her dilemma?
2. Specifically, how might Linda go about becoming an active force for positive change in the staff education department?

P/T-13-02

Topic Emphasis:	People Problems
Additional Topics:	Communication, Criticism and Discipline, Motivation

---

The Know-It-All

You are the manager of building services at James Memorial Hospital. One of the people reporting to you is Bill Douglas, the maintenance supervisor. Douglas has come to you with a complaint concerning Ed Wayne, one of his six employees. Says Douglas:

I need your help in figuring out how to handle Ed Wayne. I guess his work is okay—he isn't my best producer, but he certainly isn't the worst—but he's got such a know-it-all attitude that he drives the rest of the guys crazy.

Ed's assigned to general mechanical maintenance, but he's always trying to bust out of that and do all sorts of other things. There hasn't been a job come up in months that Ed hasn't claimed he knew how to do, and he's always trying to get his hands on everything new and different that comes along. The other guys feel that Ed is continually trying to crowd into their territory, and to make matters worse he's constantly criticizing the others and finding fault with what they do. And he's always quick with an arrogant "I-told-you-so" when someone else does something that goes wrong.

The other guys on the crew have been referring to Wayne as "the expert," but they no longer say it kiddingly. One of the fellows has even asked me to count him out when it comes to teaming him up with Wayne on jobs that take two men. I tell you, I've got to do something about this guy before his behavior destroys the whole crew's morale.

Question

What advice are you going to give Bill Douglas about dealing with know-it-all employee Wayne?

P/T-13-03

> *Topic Emphasis:*   People Problems
> *Additional Topics:*   Communication, Criticism and
>   Discipline, Motivation

The Blameless One

You are administrative supervisor in the laboratory of a 400-bed hospital. Your assistant has come to you with a complaint concerning a young man named Michaels, one of the lab's messengers. Your assistant says:

> I've just about reached the end of my rope with Michaels, and I need your advice. I can't pin him down on anything. No matter what happens or how nearly certain I am that he was involved, when it comes down to fixing responsibility he swears he was never there, he knows nothing about it, he didn't do it, or someone else is trying to make him look bad. No matter what the situation is, he's got an excuse—sometimes a really plausible one—and I can't get him to own up to anything. Even when one of the stops on his rounds gets missed he's got a long, involved story to account for it, a story I hear only if I learn about what happened and try to find out more.
>
> To hear Michaels tell it, he's never made a mistake in his life. But if I could believe him for even one minute, then I'd have to believe that the whole world around him fouls up day after day and tries to lay the blame at his feet. Tell me—what can I do about him?

Question

What advice are you going to give your assistant for dealing with the ever-blameless Michaels?

P/T-13-04

Topic Emphasis: People Problems
Additional Topics: Communication, Criticism and
Discipline, Supervisory Authority

Who Answers to Whom?

As a recently hired housekeeping supervisor at County General Hospital, Will Ross has put a great deal of effort into trying to tighten up housekeeping operations and improve staff productivity. Every day he provides each member of his crew of housekeeping aides with a work plan to follow, and he stresses that his employees are not to deviate from this plan. He has arranged his employees' work so that the workload is not unreasonable or overly demanding, but the employees have to keep working steadily to stay on schedule.

One afternoon housekeeping aide Tom Mooney was buffing a corridor in a medical/surgical unit when the unit's head nurse hurried up to him and said, "Shut that thing off and come with me. We need you to clean up a mess in room 211." Without shutting off the buffer Mooney responded, "Sorry, but I've got a schedule of things to do and only so much time to do them. Mr. Ross says I'm not to take on any extra jobs unless he tells me to."

The nurse replied, "I don't care what Mr. Ross says. Right now you're in *my* nursing unit, and when you're in my unit you'll do what I tell you to do. Now come with me."

Mooney shut off the buffer but did not move. Rather, he said, "I think we need to call Mr. Ross."

The nurse snapped, "We don't need to call anyone. Now, if you're interested in keeping your job you better do as I say."

Instructions

Decide how the foregoing incident should be handled and by whom it should be handled. In developing your tentative solution, consider the question of authority: To whose authority must Mooney ultimately respond? Why?

P/T-13-05

Topic Emphasis: People Problems
Additional Topics: Communication, Decision Making

The Voice

You are head nurse of a routine medical/surgical unit. One evening you are alone at the nursing station when a particular physician with whom you have had a number of confrontations strides up to your desk with a stormy look on his face. He says to you, "I want that nurse of yours, that Margo what's-her-face, kept out of Mr. Wilson's room. And that's final."

"Do you mean Margo Adams?"

"Whatever, the only Margo on the shift. She's gotten my patient so upset that his blood pressure's elevated."

You ask, "What's the problem?"

"Her voice! Her loud, screechy, irritating voice. Even something simple like 'Lift your hand, please' comes out like a shrill command. Two minutes in the room, and my patient is ready to climb the walls."

You respond, "Doctor, in addition to me there are only two RNs—and Mrs. Adams is one of them—to cover this entire unit on the second shift. We've been understaffed for months, and I don't see things getting any better in the near future. I don't know what I can do about Margo Adams or about her voice."

"*I* know what you can do about her," the doctor replies. "You can do exactly as I say and keep her out of Mr. Wilson's room. And if she so much as steps inside that room again I'm going to enter that fact on the patient's chart and make it a medical order that she be kept away from him."

The doctor walks away, leaving you to ponder the problem of Margo Adams's voice.

Instructions

Develop one or more possible solutions, attempting to accommodate equally, as far as possible:

1. the needs of the patient;
2. the demands of the physician (to whatever extent you feel these demands are justified);
3. the staffing requirements of your unit.

P/T-13-06

Topic Emphasis: People Problems
Additional Topics: Communication, Decision Making, Supervisory Authority

---

She Works for You

Before you were hired as business office manager at rural Jennings Hospital, the business office was run by Emma Lane. Employed by the hospital for many years, she had the title of business office supervisor until you arrived. When you were hired Lane was retained and given the title of assistant manager, but you recognized at the start that the operation was too small for the business office manager to legitimately have an assistant.

As the administrator explained the problem to you, the hospital business had bypassed Lane some years ago. Routine third-party billing requirements caused her no end of consternation, and computers were a complete mystery to her. The administrator said also, however, that Lane was such a decent person and was so well liked by others that he wished to do nothing that would upset her. You should feel no doubt, you were told, that you were hired to run the business office and that Lane's retention as assistant business office manager was simply a temporary kindness.

The problem was his, the administrator stated, and he would deal with it inside of six months. He felt that Lane would certainly "get the message" concerning the current view of her usefulness and cooperate in seeking a graceful exit. (She was not eligible for full retirement, but based on years of service she could retire early under a deferred-pension arrangement.)

More than a year has passed, and Emma Lane is still your assistant. You have seen no sign whatsoever that she may have "gotten the message." You have gone to great lengths to keep her away from tasks of any particular importance, but you have found that going about your business on a day-to-day basis is like trying to cook a full-course dinner on a tight time schedule while coping with an eager but unskilled child who is clamoring to help.

Just this week you took your concerns and frustrations to the administrator. He agreed that it certainly did not appear as though Lane was about to step down on her own. Referring to numerous instances in which her actions had caused severe problems in the business office, you put the question to the administrator point-blank: What is to be done about Emma Lane?

After considerable hemming and hawing and staring at portions of the ceiling, the administrator responded, "You've been business office manager for more than a year. That's your department. As for Mrs. Lane, she works for you. You'll have to take care of the situation as you see fit."

Instructions

1. Develop at least three alternative solutions to the problem of Emma Lane. Identify all possible advantages and disadvantages of each solution.
2. Which of your alternatives do you favor most? Why?
3. Where does the blame appear to lie; that is, how did you come to be burdened with the problem of Lane?

P/T-13-07

Topic Emphasis: People Problems
Additional Topics: Communication, Delegation, Motivation

Hairbreadth Harry

You are manager of engineering and maintenance, and in your group you have an employee you refer to (to yourself) as "Hairbreadth Harry." You took the name from a rather foolish comic book hero of years ago who was so named because he always seemed to be able to avoid calamity by the mere breadth of a hair. Your employee, also named Harry, seems to get away with almost everything and constantly avoids serious disciplinary action by the breadth of a hair.

Harry's greatest gift is the gift of gab. While generally getting into trouble through inaction, independent action, or unacceptably delayed action, Harry is generally able to talk his way out of the situation, or—and at this he excels—cast such doubt on your original instructions that he is rendered innocent by virtue of reasonable doubt. He also seems able to find a plausible reason, quite contrary to what you intended, in everything you say.

Harry's annual performance review is coming up in two weeks, and you have found it necessary to review all of the incidents you have discussed with him—and documented—over the past 12 months. You feel you have been able to remain objective about some aspects of Harry's performance; for instance, Harry has completed fewer work orders than any of your other employees, and yet his work has been the subject of a greater number of complaints than anyone else's work. His attendance record is marginal. However, Harry has come to be such a thorn in your side that you are not sure you can rightly assess him relative to the more hazily defined aspects of performance you must deal with, such as cooperation, adaptability, attitude, etc. You have, however, come to one firm conclusion regarding Hairbreadth Harry: Unless all aspects of an assignment are spelled out for him down to the last conceivable detail, Harry will find a way to slip past by the breadth of a hair.

Instructions

Develop a detailed approach to dealing with Hairbreadth Harry. In your approach you should attempt to reduce Harry's maneuvering room as much as possible, but still allow him the opportunity to correct his behavior before drastic disciplinary action is considered.

P/T-13-08

Topic Emphasis:	People Problems
Additional Topics:	Communication, Methods
	Improvement, Supervisory Authority

Your Wasteful Friend

You are one of two supervisors in the central supply department. You take your job seriously, and in light of a current economic pinch you are keenly aware of the necessity to economize whenever possible.

You are also aware that your fellow supervisor does not share your attitude and outlook and is costing the institution unnecessary expense through failure to exercise what you consider common-sense cost control. You have attempted to control costs closely because you see this as part of your job and because you believe cost control to be necessary. However, the other supervisor makes no effort to control costs and openly resists any economy-oriented changes you attempt to make.

Higher management, from the central supply manager on up, seems to be paying no attention to what is going on in the department. The other supervisor whose attitudes and actions seem constantly to frustrate your own is supposedly a close friend of yours, so you are reluctant to "blow the whistle."

Question

What approaches could you consider taking, considering that you are in a bind between the dictates of your conscience and a personal relationship?

P/T-13-09

> *Topic Emphasis:*   People Problems
> *Additional Topic:*   Decision Making

The Long-Time Employee

You have been head nurse of the east medical/surgical unit for nearly 20 years. One of your employees, a licensed practical nurse named Hilda Burns, has been part of the east unit day shift team even longer. In fact, Hilda is the only original member remaining of the crew that existed when you first took over the unit.

About six months ago Hilda Burns returned to work following an extensive illness that left her changed noticeably in a number of ways. Where once she was energetic and seemed to possess considerable stamina, now the hustle and bustle of the day shift and always being on her feet and on the move seem to wear her down rapidly. You have felt a growing concern for Hilda and for the rest of your team as well, since it has become obvious to you that Hilda is not pulling her weight on the team. The other members of your already-overworked crew are having to work extra hard to make up the difference.

Your concern reached a peak this week when three of your staff nurses came to talk with you about Hilda. Although they came to you with considerable reluctance—for Hilda has always been well liked by both staff members and patients—they were quite convinced that something had to be done both for Hilda's sake and for the sake of the department. It seems that Hilda has barely been able to accomplish half of what she should be expected to do in an eight-hour shift.

Hilda Burns knows only nursing; she has been a licensed practical nurse for all of her working life. She will not be eligible for retirement for five more years.

Question

What options might be available to you for solving the problem presented by the presence of Hilda Burns in the east medical/surgical unit?

P/T-13-10

Topic Emphasis: People Problems
Additional Topics: Communication, Rules and Policies, Supervisory Authority

---

The Requested Favor

You are head nurse of a 40-bed medical/surgical unit.

This morning one of your nurses, Mrs. Allen, came to you with a request for a "small change" in her hours of work. She asked to be permitted to start and end her shift 30 minutes earlier than scheduled. She explained that this was necessary because her husband's hours had changed (he works evenings) and she has to be home before he leaves so the children will not be unattended.

You told her that you would have to think about the request and get back to her. Your thoughts seemed to resolve into three alternatives:

1. Deny the request.
2. Grant the request.
3. Grant the request on a temporary basis, giving her some time to work out a permanent arrangement.

Questions

1. What are the advantages and disadvantages of all three?
2. Which option do you believe you should choose? Why?

P/T-13-11

> *Topic Emphasis:* People Problems
> *Additional Topics:* Communication, Rules and Policies, Supervisory Authority

---

A Next-Door Precedent

You are head nurse of 3-west, a 40-bed medical/surgical unit. This morning one of your nurses, Mrs. Dale, came to you with a problem. She had lost her regular ride to and from work. She could arrange possible transportation with one of the hospital's x-ray technicians, if she could be allowed to start and end her shift a half-hour earlier than normal.

You were about to tell Dale that the change in hours was out of the question when she said, "I don't know why I even have to ask. After all, Mrs. Johnson on 3-east lets Mrs. Allen and a couple of others juggle their hours as they please." Upon hearing this, you told Mrs. Dale you would have to do some checking and get back to her the next day.

Question

How do you believe you should respond to Dale's request? Why?

P/T-13-12

Topic Emphasis: People Problems
Additional Topics: Communication, Leadership

The Unrequested Information

One morning you were having coffee alone in the cafeteria when you were joined by Mrs. Morris, one of your employees. Morris proceeded to tell you—"in confidence, please"—that another employee, Mrs. Greely, had been passing derogatory remarks about your management style among members of the staff.

Morris proclaimed that she did not ordinarily carry stories but felt that you "had a right to know, for the good of the department."

Questions

1. Should you:
   a. thank Morris and ask her to report anything else she may hear?
   b. acknowledge her concern "for the good of the department" but tell her to bring you no further stories?
   c. thank her, ask her to say nothing to anyone else, and decide for yourself to keep an eye on Greely?
2. Why did you choose the particular answer you selected?

P/T-15-01 (R)

Topic Emphasis: Rules and Policies
Additional Topics: Communication, Leadership,
Supervisory Authority

Different Standards?

The Situation

When Janis Good was hired as evening supervisor she took the job on the understanding that hers was a Monday-through-Friday position. She was unaware that her predecessor, Mrs. Benson, had occasionally switched shifts with one of the relief supervisors and worked some weekend time. In fact, it was after several years of working in a situation in which she received only every third weekend off that Janis actively sought a nursing management position where she could work Monday through Friday only.

Janis was at the hospital for a full month before the first hint of resentment over her schedule reached her. More than once the head nurses who reported to her provided her with secondhand comments on the order of: "Some of the girls are wondering why Mrs. Good never works Saturday or Sunday." Once it even reached her ears—again secondhand—that "Mrs. Good is just too *good* to work the same hours as the rest of us."

Early in her third month Janis received a request for a meeting from Audrey Smith, a head nurse who wanted to see Janis "on behalf of all of the head nurses and several staff nurses." Janis had little doubt that the subject of the discussion would be her failure to work weekends. Janis made certain that the meeting was arranged for a time when they could talk as long as necessary without interruption.

The Role Positions

Audrey Smith. You have personally spoken with about 20 percent of the evening nursing staff, and you believe the attitudes of these people properly reflect the attitudes of all staff, that is, all of them have to take turns working weekends under the prevailing every-other-weekend-off policy, and the evening supervisor should be no different. You, Audrey, have worked every other weekend for as long as you can remember, and you consider that weekend work "goes with the territory" as far as being a nurse is concerned. The only persons in nursing you believe should work steadily Monday through Friday are the director and assistant director of nursing service and possibly the director of inservice education. These you consider to be management or top staff positions not involved with direct responsibility for patient care.

You know you will find it necessary to remind Good that Benson worked about half of the weekends, although not always in a strict every-other-weekend pattern. You believe that for the good of the evening staff you must convince Good to work her fair share of weekend time.

Janis Good. You firmly believe that shift supervisors need not always work the same hours as their employees. You are aware, of course, that a first-line supervisor should be with the group at all times; that is why head nurses work when their people work.

You also believe that the precedent apparently set by Mrs. Benson does not constitute policy and does not in any way obligate you to work weekends. You are personally opposed to working weekends, and you are certain that you would resign should you find yourself in a position of being permanently committed to working every other weekend. However, you recognize the responsibility of your position and realize there will be weekends when the head nurses will find it necessary to call you at home. Although you have strong feelings on the subject of being expected to work weekends, you are aware that an adamant stand on your part may serve to alienate you further from your employees at a time when you are striving to build acceptance and credibility.

The Meeting

Audrey Smith should begin, stating why the meeting was requested. Each party should then attempt to "sell" her position to the other. If Janis Good concedes and agrees to work weekends, she should be able to see compelling reasons for doing so. On the other hand, if Smith can be convinced that the supervisor need not work weekends she should have convincing reasons to take back to the others for whom she is speaking. However, if neither side is completely "saleable" to the other party, the two should attempt to end the meeting by arriving at a compromise solution.

P/T-15-02

> *Topic Emphasis:*   Rules and Policies
> *Additional Topics:*   Communication, People Problems

Yours, Mine, and Hours

You were recently hired as director of medical records. Among your first official acts was the hiring of an assistant director and an additional medical transcriptionist.

On the first morning of your fourth week on the job, and the second week for your two new employees, your new employees came to you with a complaint. They said they had just discovered they were working 40 hours a week, but the other employees in the department—five in all—were working only 37-1/2 hours. This was the first you had heard of anything less than a 40-hour week.

You questioned the other employees one by one. You learned that the former director of medical records, who had been there many years, hired all of these people, one by one, with promises of a 37-1/2-hour week. You told each employee, as you felt you must, that the basic workweek throughout the hospital is 40 hours, and there is no policy that states medical records is entitled to operate on the basis of a shorter workweek.

Your employees agreed that nothing was ever written down about a 37-1/2-hour week, but each claimed that this was promised orally as a condition of employment. All of them insist that the hospital is honor-bound to observe what is apparently an unwritten policy established by the former director of medical records. As one employee put it, "This place has always had a pretty good reputation as an employer, and I didn't think we had to have everything in writing."

Questions

1. What are you going to do about the predicament in which you find yourself?
2. Who else may you have to involve in the solution to your problem? Why?

P/T-15-03

Topic Emphasis: Rules and Policies
Additional Topics: Communication, People Problems, Supervisory Authority

---

Bending the Break

As supervisor of the admitting department you are also responsible for the hospital's reception area and switchboard.

Your employees, like most employees throughout the hospital, are entitled to 15-minute breaks each morning and each afternoon. Most of your employees have some flexibility as to when they can take their breaks, but two of your people, the women who work the switchboard and the reception desk, have specifically scheduled breaks because you have to provide relief while they are gone. You have no people to spare, so much of the time you personally relieve the switchboard operator and receptionist.

This was one of *those* weeks. Two people were absent most of the week, admitting activity was greater than usual, and a number of troublesome things occurred. You found it necessary to relieve Mrs. Weston, the switchboard operator, personally for morning breaks for the entire week.

On Monday and Tuesday Weston stayed away about 20 minutes. Wednesday she was gone slightly longer than 20 minutes, and on both Thursday and Friday she stayed away from the switchboard for a full half-hour. With all the work you had to do you felt you could not tolerate such long breaks, and on Friday you spoke with Mrs. Weston about her apparent habit of taking longer than the allowed time.

"I can't help it," was Weston's response. "The coffee shop is all jammed up when I take my break, and that goes for most of the morning. Two days last week I didn't get coffee at all, and another day I got it but didn't have time to drink it, all so I could be back here within 15 minutes. I know I'm entitled to only 15 minutes, but the way things are in that coffee shop I can't possibly get served, enjoy my coffee, and get back in time."

You decided to check with the receptionist, Miss Ames. Ames echoed Mrs. Weston's complaint about the crowded coffee shop and added, "What we'd really like is to have our own supply of coffee nearby. But you know as well as I do that the administrator forbids coffee pots and cups and such in the offices and public areas."

Checking with a number of your admitting department employees, you discover that most of them have learned how to take advantage of fluctuations in the morning crowd in the coffee shop. However, as far as you can determine the morning coffee break appears to be more nearly 20 minutes than 15 minutes because of waiting time.

Question

How might you go about solving the problem of having coffee available to your employees and still accomplish the morning break within the allowed time?

P/T-15-04 (R)

Topic Emphasis: Rules and Policies
Additional Topics: Communication, People Problems, Supervisory Authority

It's a Policy

The setting is an 82-bed hospital located in the center of a small city.

One day an employee of the maintenance department asked his supervisor, Mr. Mann, for an hour or two off in which to take care of some personal business. Mann agreed, and asked the employee to stop at the garden equipment shop and buy several lawnmower parts which the hospital required.

While transacting business in a local bank the employee was seen by Mr. Carter who supervised both personnel and payroll for the hospital and was in the bank on hospital business. Carter asked the employee what he was doing there and was told the visit was personal.

Upon returning to the hospital, Carter examined the employee's time card. The man had not punched out to indicate when he left the hospital. Carter noted the time the employee returned, and after the normal working day he marked the card to indicate an absence of two hours on personal business. Carter advised the administrator, Mrs. Arnold, of what he had done, citing a longstanding policy (in their dusty and infrequently used policy and procedure manual) requiring an employee to punch out when leaving the premises on personal business. The administrator agreed with Mr. Carter's action.

Carter advised Mann of the action and stated that the employee would not be paid for the two hours he was gone.

Mann was angry. He said he had told the employee not to punch out because he had asked him to pick up some parts on his trip. However, Mann conceded that the employee's personal business was probably the greater part of the trip. Carter replied that Mann had no business doing what he had done and that it was his—Mann's—poor management that caused the employee to suffer.

Mann appealed to the administrator to reopen the matter based on his claim that there was an important side to the story which she had not yet heard. Arnold agreed to hear both managers state their positions.

The Role Positions

Mann. You feel strongly that the employee should be paid for the two hours. You led him to believe he would be paid, and you also feel that in spite of the time spent on personal business it was time well used because it saved you a trip out of the hospital.

Carter. You believe in the policy, and you feel that the action sanctioned by Mann was contrary to the policy.

Arnold. Listen thoroughly to both Mann's and Carter's statements of position. Work with them to develop a mutually acceptable solution to the present problem and also to provide a way to prevent the situation from recurring.

P/T-15-05

Topic Emphasis: Rules and Policies
Additional Topics: Communication, People Problems, Supervisory Authority

---

Your Unhappy Duty

You are manager of purchasing and general stores for Ajax Memorial Hospital. In the one year you have been there you have come to know your four employees quite well. They are generally a happy, cohesive, and cooperative group, usually joking among themselves, but always getting the work done more than satisfactorily. All of them seem to give a great deal to the hospital and it is obvious to you that they care about what they are doing. A couple of them usually come in a bit early, going over their plans for the day's work over coffee before starting time, and although quitting time is 4:30 P.M., all of them generally stay 15 to 30 minutes beyond 4:30 simply to finish what they happen to be working on at quitting time. You have felt all along that you could not ask for a better group of employees.

This afternoon, however, things changed. You came in at about 3:00 P.M. from a meeting outside of the hospital to be met by four grim faces reflecting various degrees of gloom and anger. Your secretary Carol said, "The administrator is looking for you. Three calls in the last hour, in fact, although he was told you weren't due back until 3:00."

The telephone rang. Carol answered it and after a moment said, "Yes sir, he's here. He just walked in. I'll send him right up."

Without an inkling of the problem you hurried to the administrator's office where you were greeted with a stern look and a firm instruction to close the door before seating yourself.

"I want to know if you think you're running a department or a social club," the administrator snapped.

"What do you mean?"

"I was walking down the corridor near your office, and I heard an awful racket coming out of the stockroom. Laughing—so loud I could hear it a hundred feet up the corridor. I went in and found your entire staff—all four of them—eating lunch in the stockroom. Actually eating lunch in the department. Were you aware that they did so?"

"Certainly," you answered. "They've always done that. I wondered about that when I was new here, but I did enough digging to convince myself there was no rule against it."

"There are common-sense rules of behavior that I insist on. These should be sufficiently plain that they need not be written down. And eating in the department is an obvious case. Why do you think we provide a cafeteria?"

You said that you agreed as far as certain areas were concerned. For instance, you understand that it would not look good for someone to be eating lunch at the admissions desk. You believe it does not really matter in the case of your stockroom since this is a closed area never entered by patients or visitors.

"What's good for one department is good for all departments," the administrator responded. "And that goes for the coffee pot as well. I don't permit coffee pots in the departments. Your people can get their coffee in the cafeteria at specified break times just like anybody else."

Not quite biting your tongue in time you said, "There's a coffee pot in the dictating room of medical records. Of course, that's used by *doctors* as well."

Your remark triggered a few choice comments about your attitude, and you found yourself on the receiving end of a spontaneous and rather critical "performance evaluation" until just a few minutes before quitting time. Although you tried your best to defend your employees, citing their generally good-humored cooperation and flexibility, you nevertheless departed with a clear message to take back to your employees: We are running a health care organization in businesslike fashion, and that means no boisterous laughter, no eating in any part of the department, and no coffee pot.

You arrived back in your department's quarters in the lower corridor at exactly 4:30. Your four employees, grim faces and all, were the first persons in line at the time clock in the corridor. It was the first time you ever knew any of them to punch out at 4:30 on the dot.

Questions

1. Assuming you disagree with the administrator's directive, but recognizing that you are under orders to assure it is followed, how are you going to get the word across to your staff?
2. Since staff morale has already been adversely affected and you have yet to reaffirm the orders they received during the surprise visit, what can you do to try to blunt the possible demotivating effects of this turn of events?

P/T-16-01

      Topic Emphasis: Supervisory Authority
  Additional Topics: Change Management, Decision
                       Making, People Problems

The Boss Is Always the Boss

Charles Mason is controller of Morgan General Hospital. He reports to Robert Green, associate administrator for fiscal services. Green has been with the institution for a number of years, having worked his way up to controller and eventually into the top financial position which he has held for nearly five years.

Mason is the third controller reporting to Green in less than five years. He has never heard a predecessor's opinion of Green, but his own is that Green does not practice delegation to any significant extent and attempts to hang on to as much as possible of the running of the departments under his control.

Recently Morgan General entered a period of extensive change. The adoption of a new accounting system accompanied by extensive computerization changed the workload requirements in accounting. The data processing section under Mason grew in size, but general accounting and patient accounting found themselves overstaffed in terms of current needs.

Mason accepted the eventual necessity of reducing the manpower in the accounting sections; however, the new budget year was coming up and he had not yet been able to achieve this reduction through normal attrition. It looked likely that he would have to make at least two cuts by layoff or retirement. Mason knew of no one who was planning to leave in the foreseeable future, and the only person close to retirement was Ned Kline of patient accounting. Kline was nine months short of the earliest possible retirement age of 62, but had expressed his intention of working until age 65.

Along with Mason's manpower budget projections, Green requested his plans for bringing his staff down to the required level. Mason submitted two names for layoff—Brown of general accounting and Miller of patient accounting. Green responded by suggesting that Mason instead get rid of Jerry Victor and Ned Kline, both of patient accounting.

Mason did not agree, and he asked for Green's reasons. Green responded that Victor and Kline were the two least productive individuals in the department and that Kline, in addition to being marginally productive, had a chronic attitude problem. Mason disputed both of these suggested actions. In his own recommendations he had gone by straight seniority, although he was not required to do so. He considered Jerry Victor capable, and Victor was third from the bottom in seniority. Brown and Miller were the two logical ones to go on a last-in first-out basis. He generally agreed with Green about Kline's productivity and attitude, but he felt that keeping such a person around for nearly 15 years had been a management mistake and it would not be fair to get rid of him this close to retirement.

Green told Mason to do what he felt was right; he was only making suggestions.

Mason knew there was no love lost between Green and Jerry Victor; they had occasional differences on business matters, and when they communicated at all it was curtly. Mason felt that Green was using this opportunity to weed out people he did not particularly like.

One week later Green and Mason were again face to face on the same issue. Green asked if Mason had revised his recommendations. The layoffs were to take place in stages, with a pay period between individual layoffs. One from accounting had to go at the end of the current week. Mason indicated that his first choice to go was Brown.

Green reminded Mason of his earlier recommendations. He still felt that Kline and Victor should go. He pointed out that Kline would not be hurt because he had a fair amount in the retirement plan and was also known to have some real estate holdings on the side. He suggested that it did not matter that Kline desired to keep working.

On Wednesday, two days prior to the target for the first layoff, Mason prepared the termination notice for Brown. He went to Green for the necessary signature. Green refused to sign the notice. He said to Mason,

"What would you do if I gave you a direct order to lay off Jerry Victor and Ned Kline?"

"I don't know. I might refuse, or I might not," Mason said.

Green said he was going to keep the notice a while and do some thinking. Mason went away pondering what he considered to be the basic unfairness of Green's actions and wondering what he would do if it came to a confrontation.

The next day, Thursday, Green again sent for Mason. He had not signed the termination notice for Brown. Instead, before him he had termination notices for Jerry Victor and Ned Kline, the latter dated for one pay period following the former. Green had already signed them. He showed the notices to Mason and said, "I feel it's in the best interests of the finance division and the institution as a whole if these are the two people who leave. It's my belief that they are the least capable employees in the finance division. I'm sorry you chose to ignore my suggestions, and now I have to put them in the form of a direct order. You will put these two men on layoff. Sign these notices and have them delivered and talk to the people as necessary."

Instructions

Consider the primary alternatives open to Mason. He may either: (a) follow Green's instructions and lay off Victor and Kline, or (b) refuse to do so and risk the consequences. Which do you think he should do? Why?

It may help your analysis to know that Charles Mason is in his late thirties, has a bachelor's degree in accounting, and is about three-fourths of the way to a master's degree in financial management. He is married and has four children under 13 years old. During the 18 months he has been at the hospital he has taken out a five-year home-improvement loan and also purchased a second automobile. He feels that if he were forced out of work he could maintain his family's present standard of living for not more than 2 months on available resources.

P/T-16-02

Topic Emphasis: Supervisory Authority
Additional Topics: Communication, Criticism and Discipline, Decision Making

Looking for the Limits

When you accepted the position of manager of engineering and maintenance your boss, assistant administrator Peter Jackson, told you that you would not find a great deal of decision-making guidance written out in policy and procedure form. As Jackson put it, "Common sense is the overriding policy." However, Jackson cautioned you about the necessity to see him about matters involving employee discipline because the hospital was especially sensitive to union overtures in the service and maintenance areas.

Early during your third week on the job a matter arose which seemed to you to call for disciplinary action of a routine nature. Remembering Jackson's precaution, you tried to see the assistant administrator several times over a period of three days. Being unable to get Jackson and receiving no response to your messages specifically describing the situation, you went ahead and took action rather than risk losing credibility through procrastination. When you were finally able to obtain an audience with Jackson some several days later you described both the situation and the action you had taken. Jackson agreed with you, and of your apparent concern for getting to him quickly he said, "What's the big deal? As I said, common sense is the best policy and yours was a sound, common-sense decision."

When a similar situation arose some weeks later and again you could not get to Jackson although you tried to reach him several times, once again you took action. However, this time the disciplinary action involved an employee whom you later learned was a vocal informal leader of a sizable group of discontented employees. Your disciplinary action blew up in your face and provided the active union organizers with an issue which they instantly took up as a rallying point.

Jackson was furious with you, accusing you of deliberately overstepping your authority by refusing to bring such problems to his attention as he had directed.

Instructions

1. Develop a tentative approach to the determination of the limits of your decision-making authority.
2. Since the limits of your authority are ultimately those limits prescribed by your boss—and your boss is the aforementioned Peter Jackson—develop a possible approach for getting Jackson to help you define the limits of your authority.

P/T-16-03

Topic Emphasis:　Supervisory Authority
Additional Topics:　Communication, Criticism and
　　　　　　　　　　　Discipline, Hiring

He Didn't Work Out

Bill Young, an all-around mechanic and handyman, was hired by the James Memorial Hospital as supervisor of engineering and maintenance. Although he had 15 years experience in the field this was Young's first supervisory position.

Shortly after Young's arrival a maintenance helper job became available. This was an important job because of a number of necessary upkeep tasks which had to be performed, and Bill Young recognized the need to fill this job as soon as possible. On first receiving the departing helper's resignation, Young contacted the personnel department and asked them to locate several candidates for him to interview.

Young's immediate supervisor, assistant administrator Peter Jackson, chose to sit in on the interviews, giving as his reason Young's newness to management. Jackson indicated that since Young had never interviewed or hired before he should be assisted in the process.

Young and Jackson jointly interviewed five candidates. Of the five, two appeared to be reasonably qualified for the job. One of these was a young man named Simmons who was employed at the hospital in the dishroom of the dietary department. The other was a young man named Kelly who had not worked recently but had had several months of building-and-grounds experience on the custodial staff of a school.

Following the interviews Young expressed his desire to hire Simmons from the dishroom because he appeared to have the aptitude and ability and exhibited a strong desire to better himself. However, Jackson disagreed with Young, told Young he could do the hiring "the next time a job opened," and made the decision to hire Kelly for the job.

As the 30-day probation period progressed it became increasingly evident to Bill Young that Kelly was not shaping up as a satisfactory employee. Even extending every benefit of the doubt, which he did because of Kelly being "the boss's choice," he could conclude only that they would not benefit from having Kelly as a permanent employee.

On the twenty-eighth day of Kelly's employment Bill Young went to see Jackson. He had kept Jackson advised of Kelly's poor progress and lack of response to suggestions, so it was no surprise to Jackson when Young said they should let Kelly go and start all over again.

"Okay," was Jackson's reply, "let Kelly go."

Young hesitated, wondering for a moment if he should say anything, and finally said to Jackson, "I don't believe *I* should let him go. I didn't hire him."

"He's your employee," Jackson responded. "*You* get rid of him."

Questions

1. Do you believe Jackson shirked responsibility by ordering Young to get rid of Kelly? Why, or why not?
2. In what other ways—at least two are possible—could this situation have been more equitably handled?
3. What effect is the Kelly incident likely to have on the future relationship between Young and Jackson?

P/T-16-04

Topic Emphasis:	Supervisory Authority
Additional Topics:	Communication, Criticism and Discipline, Rules and Policies

---

Out on a Limb

One winter morning John Moran, manager of engineering and maintenance for Community Hospital, told maintenance employee Robert Best to shovel the snow from the sidewalks leading to the main entrance.

Best refused. Initially he pleaded health, saying he was too weak to do such heavy work. Moran said he knew of no illness or disability on Best's part and knew there was nothing in the man's employment record indicating the need for restricting physical effort. Best then changed the nature of his objections, saying that since there was nothing in his job description requiring him to shovel snow he did not have to do it. Moran pointed out the job description phrase, "And all other duties as directed by supervision." However, this did not satisfy Best, and he again refused to shovel the snow.

Moran and Best had almost come head to head on a similar matter once in the past; Best refused to do something assigned to him, but while he and Moran were arguing the case the necessity to perform the disputed task disappeared unexpectedly. At that time Moran told Best that he could consider himself as having received a verbal warning, and that if such a thing occurred again it would be written up as a case of insubordination and taken up the chain of command for disposition. (Community Hospital had no policy governing the use of written warnings. However, Moran chose to cover his tracks with letters which were reviewed with offending employees before being placed in their personnel files.)

Moran wrote up the snow-shoveling refusal as a case of insubordination and requested a meeting with the assistant administrator. He asked that Best be present at the meeting.

At the meeting Moran presented the letter, described the situation, and recommended that Best be discharged for insubordination. The assistant administrator listened, then advised Best that he would not be fired and sent him back to work with a mild reprimand (back to his regular job, *not* to shoveling snow).

After Best had left, the assistant administrator said to Moran, "You'd only be making a lot of noise without making it stick. Remember, Best's uncle is on the hospital board."

Moran left the assistant administrator's office feeling extremely bitter about the situation. This was, he reflected, the second time in recent months that the assistant administrator refused to back him in a disciplinary action. And the previous occasion had not even involved an employee with board connections.

Questions

1. What approach should Moran take with his immediate boss, the assistant administrator, in developing an understanding on matters of employee discipline?
2. What options are available to Moran the next time he encounters a situation in which he believes an employee should be disciplined?

P/T-16-05

Topic Emphasis:	Supervisory Authority
Additional Topics:	Communication, Decision Making, People Problems

Pleasant Dreams

You are head nurse on nights in a medical/surgical unit. For several months you have had a problem with a staff nurse whose performance you consider unsatisfactory. You have reprimanded her several times for sleeping on the job, and you have reached the point where you no longer feel you can simply scold her for her conduct. (Your hospital has a policy governing written warnings. Verbal warnings are unlimited; at your discretion you may deliver as many as you feel are necessary.)

For a written warning to be official and entered in an employee's personnel file, it must be agreed to and signed by nursing management and administration. You have issued the offending nurse two written warnings; both have cleared through nursing, and the offending nurse was counseled by the director of nursing service. However, you can go no further without administrative backing, and there has been no follow-up from administration. Meanwhile, the employee continues to be a problem.

Question

Assuming you consider the problem severe enough to constitute a risk to the patients under your care, what are you going to do about the unsatisfactory employee?

P/T-16-06

Topic Emphasis: Supervisory Authority
Additional Topics: Communication, Delegation

Who's the Boss?

General maintenance man Don Kendall had a few regularly scheduled tasks he performed without direction, but on most days he depended upon maintenance supervisor Sam Walters for most of his work. It was such a day that Friday when Walters said to Kendall at the beginning of the shift, "Don, I want you to paint the small conference room next to the administrator's office today. We just found out that the new furniture is coming tomorrow, so it's important to get it done today."

Don went to work on the conference room as told. However, shortly before lunch he was interrupted by Charles Johnson, the manager of engineering and maintenance and Sam Walters's boss, who said, "Drop what you're doing, Kendall. I've got a job for you."

Johnson explained, "I'm tired of getting complaints about the lighting in admitting and medical records. I want you to go through both departments and replace all fluorescent tubes that are weak or out. Also, clean all the reflectors; shine them up good. The whole job should take maybe two or three hours."

Don told Johnson what Walters had said about getting the conference room painted so the new furniture could be moved in the next day. Johnson heard him out but did not alter his instructions concerning admitting and medical records. Johnson simply said, "Get going on those lights. When Walters catches up with you, tell him to see me."

It was mid-afternoon before supervisor Walters discovered that the work on the conference room had stopped before lunch. When he finally found Kendall, which he had to do by asking several people if they had seen the maintenance man, he asked, "What's going on?"

"Mr. Johnson said I had to do this right away," answered Kendall. "I'm supposed to tell you to see him."

Instructions

1. The foregoing illustrates a fundamental error in management practice. Identify and describe this error.
2. Describe the potential effects of this specific incident on manager Johnson, supervisor Walters, and maintenance man Kendall.

P/T-16-07

Topic Emphasis:	Supervisory Authority
Additional Topics:	Communication, Leadership, People Problems

---

One Boss Too Many

The engineering and maintenance groups of Memorial Hospital are headed by three first-line supervisors. These supervisors and a department secretary report directly to a manager of engineering and maintenance who in turn reports to the director of environmental services.

The institution is in the midst of a prolonged period of growth and expansion. Almost weekly some organizational unit or other is being relocated to new quarters or drastically rearranged within its original area. The institution promises to be in a chronic state of change for some time to come, with much extra effort required by engineering and maintenance as numerous areas are opened, renovated, or rearranged.

The position of director of environmental services was created at the start of this period of major change. The incumbent was hired specifically for his apparent ability to get a new operation "up and running" through active involvement of personnel at all levels.

The director was quick to discover that his immediate subordinate, the manager of engineering and maintenance, came across as a man of considerable inertia who moved slowly, was reluctant to change, and usually defended "the way we've always done things."

Although the manager had long-time contacts with the three supervisors, the director began avoiding the manager and dealing directly with the first-line supervisors. Most things, however, found their way back to the manager who would then take action or give instructions contrary to what the director had done.

After several weeks in this mode of operation one of the first-line supervisors summed things up as follows: "We now have two bosses, and they're opposed to each other on everything. What one decides, the other reverses; what one puts together, the other tears apart. They can't even agree on anything as basic as the obvious need for disciplinary action. How do we go about maintaining effectiveness in dealing with our employees, and how do we prevent morale and efficiency from going straight down the drain?"

Instructions

Deal with the question posed by the supervisor in the final paragraph of the case. Based on what you believe to be sound management practice, develop an approach which the three supervisors might take. State any assumptions you may have to make, and fully explain the reasons for your recommended approach.

P/T-16-08 (R)

Topic Emphasis:	Supervisory Authority
Additional Topics:	Communication, People Problems, Personal Effectiveness

The Split Secretary

Background

Kate James, the hospital's manager of staff development, and Dan Young, the director of public relations and development, share a secretary. It is the job of the secretary, Ann Wilson, to provide all necessary clerical support for both staff development and public relations. This arrangement is new. Although Kate James has been involved in education at the hospital for some time, until recently she was looking after inservice education for nursing exclusively. Dan Young is new to public relations and development, which only recently became a full-time function. Ann Wilson is likewise new to the hospital.

The Role Positions

Kate James. It is Thursday, and you have had a terribly busy week so far. It has taken you all morning to develop the remainder of the handout material you need for the class you are scheduled to conduct at 8:30 Friday morning. You have been concerned about getting this stuff finished by noon because it should take Ann all afternoon to do the typing and duplicating. You realize this is cutting things pretty close, but the demands on your time have been extremely heavy and you simply were not able to get it ready sooner. You are confident, however, that Ann can have everything typed in three hours or so and with you proofreading and assisting in duplicating and collating, everything should be done by the end of the day. As you approach Ann's desk with your hands full of material you encounter Dan Young. He also appears to be approaching Ann.

Dan Young. You have been thinking it is a bit unfair for you to be expected to outline a proposed new endowment fund campaign for the board of directors during your third week on the job, especially on such short notice. The administrator gave you the assignment Monday morning and you have been working day and night since then. It is now Thursday, nearly noon, and the board meeting at which you must appear is tonight. You finally have everything assembled in handwritten draft form, but you feel it will take most of the afternoon for Ann to type it and assemble it for distribution to the board.

On your way to Ann's office you encounter Kate James. Noticing the pile of papers in Kate's hands, your first thought is that if Kate is taking some work to Ann it will simply have to wait.

Ann Wilson. After only a brief period of working jointly for Kate James and Dan Young, your most fervent wish is that you could get more advance notice of what you are expected to do and when it must be completed. You feel that you have been relatively successful in juggling their requirements and demands, but you know this cannot last forever. Someday soon, you fear, you are going to be put in a bind when the two of them both want something important at the same time.

Kate James and Dan Young approach you simultaneously. They both have papers in their hands. You are wondering if this is the day when the "big squeeze" is going to hit.

Instructions

The persons taking the roles of Kate James, Dan Young, and Ann Wilson are to work their way through the situation and reach some form of agreement which will reasonably accommodate the needs of both staff development and public relations. However, consideration should extend well beyond the solution of the immediate problem; steps should be taken to minimize the likelihood of such a "crunch" descending on them again. Throughout the role play each supervisor must recognize that although he or she has a certain amount of authority over the secretary, the secretary is also organizationally responsive to the other supervisor as well. The supervisors should also recognize that although the problem is essentially theirs because it stems from their work patterns, the secretary is unavoidably part of the problem. As part of the problem she should be considered as a potentially valuable contributor to the solution.

GROUP 2

Primary Focus: PEOPLE
Secondary Focus: SELF

P/S-02-01 (R)

Topic Emphasis: Communication
Additional Topics: Criticism and Discipline, People Problems, Personal Effectiveness

You Goofed

Recently the hospital acquired its second administrative assistant in the person of Phillip West. Phil had no experience in health care; however, in another environment he had established an impressive track record as a trouble-shooter of management problems.

One of Phil's first assignments was to examine the structure of the pathology department and suggest ways to correct certain organizational weaknesses. He spent a great deal of time speaking with and listening to the people who ran pathology. He recognized that he had a great deal to absorb, since he was unfamiliar with hospital operations even to the point of lacking knowledge of medical terminology.

After about four weeks Phil submitted a preliminary report to administration and the director of pathology. In the second paragraph of his report he had committed a grievous error in terminology: Following the reasoning that if persons practicing medicine in the hospital comprised the medical staff, then persons working in the department of pathology made up "the pathological staff."

When the director of pathology, unhappy with the idea of having his department studied in the first place, read the report he got no farther than "pathological staff" in the second paragraph. He flew into a near rage. Going immediately to the administrator, the director demanded that this "piece of junk" be scrapped and Phil be kept out of his department.

The administrator quickly realized that the director had not read beyond the second paragraph of the report. The administrator felt there were a number of sound ideas in the report, but also felt that Phil had committed a few errors due to his lack of familiarity with the hospital setting. Not easily calmed, the pathology director insisted that Phil be disciplined severely.

The administrator agreed only that Phil had to be "set straight on a few things."

After the director had left the office and the administrator had briefly considered the situation, Phil arrived. The administrator dropped a copy of the report on the desk and said, "You really dropped a bomb in the lab, Phil."

Instructions

Phillip West. You sincerely believe the matter of terminology to be of minor importance. You are convinced that the director's anger is simply a screen to keep attention away from the real problem—severe inefficiency in the department of pathology.

Administrator. You will concede that Phil uncovered some potential trouble spots in pathology, but you also believe that Phil's work will lack credibility as long as he does not "speak the language."

Together. Keeping in mind the extent to which the pathology director has been antagonized, develop a solution which accounts for:

- any criticism Phil may deserve;
- the correction of Phil's apparent shortcomings;
- some means of getting the pathology director to examine the true contents of the report.

P/S-02-02

Topic Emphasis: Communication
Additional Topics: Delegation, Personal Effectiveness, Supervisory Authority

---

Hands Off

In the year since you became housekeeping supervisor you have become increasingly unhappy with your relationship with your boss, Harry Smith, the manager of building services. In fact, Smith seems indifferent to you much of the time and even seems to go out of his way to avoid having contact with you. You do not believe that Smith treats all of his subordinate supervisors in the same fashion, so you nurture the impression that Smith either plays favorites among the supervisors or harbors a particular dislike for you.

You cannot understand why you do not have a satisfactory relationship with Smith. You cannot conceive of a higher manager who might not have had a hand in appointing his subordinate supervisors, and although you originally received word of your promotion from assistant administrator Peter Jackson at a time when Harry Smith was on sick leave you had always assumed that Smith had had an active role in your selection.

On Monday of this week you had to take immediate action on a matter of discipline which could have far-reaching implications. You fully realized the sensitive nature of the problem, and you were well aware of the importance of bringing Smith up to date on the matter and securing his backing and support. However, it was two days before you could manage to get a few minutes of your boss's time, and when you did get his attention for a short while he refused to back you in your decision. After you had described the problem and what you had done about it Smith said to you, "I've already picked up pieces of the problem via the rumor mill instead of getting it from you, and that should never happen. Besides, I'm not in favor of your decision and I'm not about to stick my neck out by sanctioning your action."

Your accumulated frustration finally coming to the surface, you said, "I've been trying to reach you since it happened, but it seems you're not the most available person in this hospital. And this is at least the third time your backing hasn't been there when I needed it. Don't you believe in supporting the supervisors who work for you?"

"Yes, most of the time," snapped Smith. "Except in your case. You weren't my choice as supervisor, and I had nothing to do with your appointment. I don't like having someone else's choice shoved down my throat."

You asked, "What do you mean someone else's choice?"

"Your promotion was strictly Jackson's idea. I had recommended another person, but Jackson went ahead and gave you the job when I was on sick leave. So I'm keeping hands off. You can run your department any way you want as far as I'm concerned. Just don't drag me into your problems."

That is where you now stand. Your initial impulse is to pay a visit to Peter Jackson. However, you recall from experience that Jackson is fully as difficult to get a few minutes with as is Smith.

Questions

1. Now that you know where you stand with Smith, what might you consider saying or doing to attempt to improve the relationship?
2. How will present circumstances influence your behavior in regard to marginal or sensitive decisions in the near future?
3. What hazards are inherent in a direct approach to assistant administrator Peter Jackson?
4. In what ways could Smith's "hands-off" policy be made to work in your favor?

P/S-05-01

Topic Emphasis: Delegation
Additional Topics: Communication, Leadership, People
Problems

The Independent Employee

Maintenance supervisor Jim Wood often felt that he had his hands full getting electrical repairman Bob Trent to follow his instructions. A case in point: On Monday of this week Wood realized that the laboratory air conditioning unit was due for its semiannual servicing and inspection, a task which either Bob Trent or one other repairman usually accomplished. He further realized that if this job was not done by the end of Wednesday it was not likely to get done for some time; some new equipment was scheduled to arrive on Thursday, and Trent's fellow repairman would be gone on vacation the following week.

Wood customarily tried to assign Trent two or three days' work at a time, since once he was under way Trent could usually be found (or not found, as was often the case) just about any place in the building tackling his assigned tasks—and often a number of unassigned tasks—in seemingly random order. Wood gave Trent the maintenance file on the laboratory air conditioner and said, "You don't necessarily have to do this first, but I'd like you to take care of it today or tomorrow. In any case it has to be finished by noon Wednesday."

Trent simply shrugged and took the file.

Wood did not see Bob Trent again until the Thursday morning coffee break. Neither had the laboratory air conditioner crossed Wood's mind until the sight of Trent reminded him of it. He approached Trent and asked, "Any trouble with the lab air conditioner?"

"Haven't done it yet," Trent said.

Wood felt a flash of anger. His schedule was blown, and it would be days, if not weeks, before the department could recover.

"Why not?" asked Wood. "I specifically told you that it had to be finished by noon Wednesday."

"I almost got started on it," said Trent, "but the assistant administrator collared me and told me he wanted the fan-coil unit in his office fixed right away. I had to tear the whole thing down to do it, but I figured that was more important than the air conditioner in the lab."

Wood felt a sense of frustration. He said, "Bob, this is the fourth time— at least—that I can think of when I've told you specifically to do something and you went and decided that something else was more important. Just what do you think I mean when I delegate something to you, anyway?"

Trent shrugged and said, somewhat defensively, "I don't know, Mr. Wood, but I figure when I see something that's more important than what I'm doing at the moment I better take care of it. Anyway, if the lab air conditioner was so all-fired important how come you didn't say anything about it until now?"

Instructions

Analyze the foregoing occurrence of incomplete delegation, criticizing the conduct of both supervisor and employee as necessary. Spell out those steps which you believe Jim Wood should take in the future to assure that Bob Trent does not decide that other tasks are "more important" than duties specifically assigned by Wood.

P/S-05-02

Topic Emphasis:	Delegation
Additional Topics:	Communication, Motivation, People Problems

---

"It's His Job, Not Mine"

As unit manager of the x-ray department you have found that your workload has been increasing to the point where you need help with certain nonmanagerial duties. One of the first tasks that comes to mind for delegation is your monthly statistical report. The creation of the report is fairly easy, but gathering the data is time-consuming.

You select an employee to do the report, and you provide the necessary instructions. You were sure to select an employee you believed capable of doing a decent job and who had sufficient time available. The person you chose expressed no feelings for or against doing the report.

Two days after assigning the task you find that the report has not yet been started. You remind the employee, but the assigned person still does not seem to be in any particular hurry to get the work done.

Shortly thereafter you accidentally overhear a portion of a conversation in which the employee to whom you have assigned the report says to another employee: ". . . his lousy statistics, and I think he ought to do it himself. After all, it's in *his* job description, not mine."

Instructions

1. Determine what might have been done incorrectly in delegating the report to the employee.
2. Decide what you can do to try to correct the employee's attitude as revealed in the final paragraph of the case.

P/S-13-01

Topic Emphasis:	People Problems
Additional Topics:	Communication, Criticism and Discipline, Delegation

---

"Why Should I?"

You are unit manager of the clinical laboratory. You have 22 employees reporting to you.

You feel that you have a comfortable working relationship with all of your employees except one. The single employee in question, a licensed laboratory technologist, continually gives you a hard time regarding assignments. Whenever you give this person a task that is not part of her regular routine or does not appear explicitly in her job description, her response is: "Why should I? That's not part of my job."

In one recent exchange you found yourself responding angrily, "Because I said so, that's why!" You immediately discovered that this response not only failed to get results, but it also generated considerable hostility.

Question

How are you going to deal with this employee?

P/S-16-01

Topic Emphasis: Supervisory Authority
Additional Topics: Communication, Leadership, People
Problems

Breach of Confidence

Mary French is head nurse of a medical/surgical unit. Her close friend, June Ross, is head nurse of a similar unit located on the floor directly above Mary's unit.

One day following their normal shift, an obviously troubled June sought Mary's advice as both a head nurse and a friend relative to a delicate situation existing in June's unit. Mary and June held a lengthy conversation in a private corner of the nurses' lounge. June asked Mary to keep the matter confidential.

Their conversation was observed, but not heard, by their immediate supervisor, Miss Jenkins. The following morning Jenkins visited Mary in her unit and said, "I saw you talking with June yesterday. I've gotten a growing sense that something is wrong on her floor, and I think it has gotten to a point where it's affecting her unit's performance. Please tell me about it."

Mary's response was, "The matter is largely personal, and I would be violating a confidence if I told you."

Jenkins responded, "Anything that affects nursing performance affects patient care whether it's personal or not. I want to be told."

Questions

1. How should Mary respond to Jenkins?
2. What steps should Mary consider if Jenkins is not satisfied with a "simple answer" and refuses to let the matter rest?

P/S-17-01

Topic Emphasis:	Time Management
Additional Topics:	Communication, Personal Effectiveness, Supervisory Authority

---

How Time Flies

You are the business office manager at Community Hospital. At 9:00 this morning your boss, the controller, called you into his office for—as he put it—"a little chitchat, ten minutes or so, on where we stand on getting the new procedure manuals done." You scooped up the proper papers and went into his office, bracing yourself because you knew how frustrating these sessions could be.

When you entered and seated yourself the controller was shuffling through the clutter on his desk looking for a particular document. At the same time he found the document he also found a pink telephone message slip apparently left over from the previous day. He said, "Oh-oh, should have done this yesterday. Excuse me just a minute."

The "minute" turned out to be a quarter of an hour as he transacted a bit of business and engaged in some social conversation. You fidgeted, wondering as you always did at such times whether you should simply get up and leave and return when he was free.

You were perhaps five minutes under way with the true subject of your meeting when the telephone rang. Your boss answered it himself, although his secretary was in her usual place. This time it was fully ten minutes before you could return to the subject of the meeting. Before you concluded your business, your boss had taken two more calls and made a brief additional call for something which he had "just remembered."

When at last you were finished to the boss's satisfaction you rose to leave. He rose also, reaching for his empty coffee cup. On the way out of his office he glanced at his watch and said, "Wow, 10:00 o'clock already. Time sure flies."

You made no comment. You were well aware that the pile of work on your desk had gotten no smaller while you were tied up for a full hour trying to accomplish about ten minutes' worth of true work.

Questions

1. What assumptions about the value of *your* time and *his* time are implicit in the boss's behavior?
2. What can you possibly do or attempt to do to encourage your boss to show more respect for your working time?

GROUP 3

Primary Focus: TASK
Secondary Focus: PEOPLE

T/P-01-01

Topic Emphasis: Change Management
Additional Topics: Communication, Decision Making, Motivation

---

The New Dictating Machines

"We got a fantastic deal on these minicassette dictating machines," said the purchasing agent, "and because of the number we went for we got the transcribing units way below cost."

"Perhaps you should have taken this up with me," said administrative secretary Sharon Smith. "I could have made some useful suggestions. What made you decide on these, anyway?"

"For one thing, they're what Mr. Miller, the associate administrator, wanted, and he's my boss—remember? In fact, Miller is the one who referred the salesman to me."

"Well, maybe you and Mr. Miller should have looked a little further. You know Polly is our very best typist, and Polly won't touch these minicassettes for anything."

"Why not?"

"She says she prefers the old belt machines. She's always worked with belts, and enough belts are still being used that she latches on to all of them and leaves the little tapes for the others to do. And don't forget, we still have a couple of those old disc machines floating around. Polly will do the discs if I ask her specifically, but Eleanor usually handles those."

"The belt machines are over the hill," the purchasing agent said. "They break down frequently, they're tough to get parts for, and we have to wait days at a time for service. The disc machines are even worse. Antiques!"

"Speaking of being bad," said Sharon, "I understand the minicassette transcribing machines have a very high frequency of repair. The recorders are supposedly pretty good, but not the transcribers. Did you check this out at all?"

"Certainly I did. The salesman referred me to a local firm which uses their complete system. I talked with their purchasing agent, and he was quite satisfied with the units."

"Well, that may be so, but you still should have checked with us. We're the ones who have to use them, you know."

"I did, in a way. I talked with two or three of the people who dictate, and I spoke with two people in the pool about the transcribing units."

"Is that all? That's just a small percentage of the people around here who will probably be using those units."

Somewhat defensively the purchasing agent said, "Look, I don't have time to run around and talk to everybody in the whole hospital about something like this. I looked at a lot of different equipment, and I'm satisfied that we got the best deal available. And if you're going to look at it that way, then I guess you're just stuck with them."

"Yes, I guess we are," Sharon said without enthusiasm.

Questions

1. What was wrong about the way the new units were selected and introduced?
2. Should—or could—the purchase of the units have been approached differently? How?
3. Assuming the hospital is indeed "stuck with" the new units, what can be done to increase the likelihood of their acceptance?

T/P-01-02

Topic Emphasis:	Change Management
Additional Topics:	Communication, Leadership, Motivation

Surprise!

On Monday morning when the business office employees arrived at the hospital they immediately noticed the apparent absence of the office manager. This was not unusual; the manager was frequently absent on Monday. However, he rarely failed to call his department when he would not be there—but on this day he still had not called by noon.

Shortly after lunch the two working supervisors in the business office were summoned to the administrator's office. There they were told that the office manager was no longer employed by the hospital. They, the two supervisors, were told to look after things for the current week and that a new manager, already secured, would be starting the following Monday. All the supervisors were told about the new manager was that it was somebody from outside of the hospital.

The supervisors were not told whether the former manager resigned or was discharged, nor were they told whether anyone within the department had been considered as a replacement.

Questions

1. What was right or wrong about the manner in which the change in business office manager was made?
2. What would you suppose to be the attitudes of the business office staff upon hearing of the change?
3. With what attitudes do you suppose the staff will receive the new manager?
4. In what other ways might this change have been approached?

T/P-01-03

> *Topic Emphasis:* Change Management
> *Additional Topics:* Communication, Methods Improvement, Motivation

---

Answers . . . ?

You are the hospital's business office manager. Among several groups within your responsibility is the billing department which is made up of a supervisor and eight clerks.

You have just made a detailed study of certain problems in the operation of the billing department. The study suggests a number of improvements, all developed with the participation of the supervisor and her clerks, aimed at improving total operations.

However, the study also suggests that part of the problem stems from the fact that the supervisor, who is located in a room apart from her staff, does not have visual control of the group's activities. Her present office is about 75 feet down the corridor from the department, and the intervening space is filled with washrooms and air conditioning equipment. Your study recommends that the supervisor's office be relocated, and there is space in the staff area for a small, semienclosed office.

With few reservations the supervisor agrees to all of the proposed changes except the relocation. She has stated in no uncertain terms that she will not be moved again; her whole group has been moved twice during the past ten years. She has threatened to resign if moved; however, she had made the threat of resignation numerous times during her ten-plus years of employment.

You believe that the agreed-upon improvements—there are some 20 specific recommendations—are necessary to the functioning of the group, and you also feel there would be considerable value in relocating the supervisor. It is up to you to decide upon an approach to the problem.

Instructions

Develop several possible approaches to avoiding or overcoming the supervisor's resistance to the relocation of her office. Keeping in mind your primary objective of improving the operation of the department, evaluate each possible solution according to the following criteria:

a. likely *cost* of implementation;
b. *fairness* to all employees; and
c. *consistency* with sound management practice and with the objectives of the organization.

T/P-01-04

Topic Emphasis:	Change Management
Additional Topics:	Communication, Methods
	Improvement, People Problems

In Need of Improvement

You are an administrative staff specialist newly hired by the hospital to act as an in-house management engineer.

Your first assignment is to conduct a study of work methods and staff in central supply. This department was singled out for study because:

- The manager, a registered nurse who has held the job for more than 25 years, has requested two more aides although her staff is already one person larger than that of another area hospital of equal size.
- There has been a recent sharp upturn in the use of disposables.
- A number of storage shelves appear to be filled to overflowing with infrequently used items.
- The department issues frequent rush orders to obtain needed items that have run completely out.
- Observed conditions in the department include an overcrowded storage area, a seemingly inadequate decontamination area, and a grossly oversized processing area referred to by most employees as "the ballroom."

On your initial visit to the department the first thing the manager says to you is: "So you're the one who's going to tell us what we're doing wrong?" Her tone is none too friendly.

Instructions

Develop a proposed approach to a complete study of the department, including a "sales pitch" intended to win the manager's cooperation and support, specifying what should be done and why it should be done.

T/P-01-05

Topic Emphasis: Change Management
Additional Topics: Communication, Motivation, People Problems

"I Used To Run This Unit"

For several years Community Hospital had difficulty obtaining enough registered nurses to fill all necessary nursing positions. As a result, for nearly two years the head nurse of medical/surgical unit 2-A was Ms. Adams, a licensed practical nurse (in spite of state code requirements to the contrary).

Recently a registered nurse, Mrs. Williams, was hired as head nurse of 2-A. Adams, no longer designated head nurse, remained with the unit as one of the staff. Although the change was clearly a demotion for Adams in terms of leaving supervision, she did not suffer financially. In fact, she had recently received a pay increase in conjunction with a favorable performance evaluation. Her increase placed her near the top of the pay range for a licensed practical nurse, but still left a small amount of room for her to advance financially.

Adams has said little about the change, and Williams, aware of the potentially troublesome situation, has had considerable difficulty attempting to "read" Adams's reaction. Adams's very few comments can be summarized as follows:

> I can see why the hospital prefers a registered nurse in charge of every unit; however, I ran this unit successfully for nearly two years. All of my evaluations have been good, I've gotten regular raises, and there has never been any real criticism of my work. When I was given the position it was never suggested to me that it would be anything but permanent.

Questions

1. How might Williams go about directing instructions to Adams in such a way as to minimize the chances of hard feelings?
2. What likely past actions or oversights contributed to the problem?
3. If Adams becomes resentful to the point of being uncooperative, what alternatives may be open to Williams?

T/P-04-01

Topic Emphasis:	Decision Making
Additional Topics:	Communication, Methods Improvement, People Problems

---

Deciding under Pressure

You are director of nursing in a 200-bed hospital. Several times during the past few months the emergency room supervisor has mentioned to you that the emergency room was getting steadily busier and she had to have more help. Her requests have never been more specific than "more help," nor have they been strongly stated. You have not yet looked into the situation.

However, on Monday of this week the supervisor came to you and said, "We need one more nurse and more clerical help *now*. I'm tired of waiting and tired of being overworked, and if something isn't done this week you can find yourself a new supervisor."

Instructions

1. There are several decisions you could make, depending on what you consider to be the real problem. List several possible "solutions" and enumerate the advantages and disadvantages of each.
2. The pressure referred to in the title has placed you in a trap. Describe this trap, and explain why it is indeed a trap.

T/P-07-01 (E)

Topic Emphasis: Hiring
Additional Topics: Communication, Rules and Policies,
Supervisory Authority

Who Hires?

Within your institution a controversy has long been shaping up between the director of personnel on one hand and several supervisors, managers, and department heads on the other. The disagreement involves the employment process and a question of who actually does the hiring.

All members of management generally agree that personnel locates and screens job candidates and provides applicants who fit the jobs' broad requirements to the departments for interviewing. The controversy first developed when the personnel director said *no* to the hiring of two applicants whom individual supervisors wanted to employ. Disagreement intensified when the personnel department "hired" a job candidate and sent her to a supervisor who had found her unsatisfactory during a personal interview.

Instructions

1. Develop a set of guidelines describing what you believe the true personnel department role in hiring should be.
2. Develop a parallel set of guidelines describing the role of the individual supervisor in hiring.
3. The personnel activity is frequently described as a "staff function." Describe how this differs from a so-called "line function," and decide what this difference says about the position of the personnel function in an organization.

T/P-10-01

Topic Emphasis:	Meetings
Additional Topics:	Communication, Motivation, People Problems

---

The Weekly Staff Meeting

There are 15 people in your department. It nas been your practice to hold a weekly staff meeting at 3:00 P.M. each Wednesday. Rather, we should say you *attempt* to hold it at 3:00 P.M. because about half of your people are more than five minutes late, and a couple of them are usually late by fifteen minutes or more.

You have made repeated announcements about being there on time, but to no avail. Come Wednesday at 3:00 P.M. you usually find yourself and the same six or seven punctual attendees present and waiting for the latecomers.

Question

Without turning at once to disciplinary action (which should always be the last resort), what can you do to encourage punctuality in attending your staff meetings?

T/P-11-01

Topic Emphasis: Methods Improvement
Additional Topics: Change Management,
Communication

The Preadmission Problem

The hospital has been experiencing difficulty with the retrieval of medical records because many admissions have been made without advance information being given to the admitting department. In other words, the hospital has not been informed in advance of many elective admissions. Nevertheless, the admitting physicians request the medical records of people who have previously been patients at the hospital, and such records should be available at the time a patient is admitted.

Since it is not known in advance that a particular patient will be admitted, each admission necessitates a special trip to medical records to check for records of previous admissions. This causes many unnecessary trips to the medical record department during the day shift. During the second and third shifts the nurses must pull the records (if records are to be made available at all). Consequently, records for patients admitted on the second and third shifts are often not available the following morning when the doctors arrive.

There were past attempts at establishing preadmission forms, but all such procedures have broken down. Presently there is no preadmission procedure in operation at the hospital.

Instructions

Using any approach you wish, develop and outline a system or procedure for solving the preadmission problem.

T/P-11-02

Topic Emphasis: Methods Improvement
Additional Topics: Change Management,
Communication, Leadership

The Troubled Department

The medical record department of your hospital is staffed with seven persons whose titles and duties are as follows:

a. Manager—department supervision, disease coding, and monthly reporting.
b. Secretary—discharge and service analysis, processing of information requests.
c. Clerk A—admissions recording, readmissions record retrieval, and daily census.
d. Clerk B—delinquency reporting, maintenance of physicians' files of incomplete charts, general filing, and routine clerical work.
e. Clerk C—microfilming, disease indexing.
f. Transcriptionist A—typing of dictated reports, delivery of reports, and insertion into charts.
g. Transcriptionist B—same as transcriptionist A.

Attention has been focused on this department for a number of reasons:

a. Transcription continually experiences a sizable backlog of dictation.
b. A backlog of disease coding has grown to unmanageable proportions.
c. Information requests from attorneys and insurance companies are being answered from 60 to 120 days after receipt.
d. Eighty percent of staff physicians regularly exceed the legal two-week limit on chart completion.
e. Clerk A is regularly caught up on current work and partially idle; the secretary and clerk B have been unable to catch up on their work for a number of months.

Standard task-time data published by various organizations suggest that the record department of this size hospital should operate smoothly with five to six persons, so assume that the present staff should be more than adequate. Also, surveys have revealed that medical record cost per patient day in this hospital is 10 percent to 15 percent high.

Instructions

1. Assume that each of the reasons for focusing attention on the department stated above is a *symptom* of some greater problem. For each symptom determine what *could be* the problem behind it; state *why*—

other than simply pointing to the symptom—you think the problem could indeed *be* a problem; and suggest an approach to solving the problem.

2. Identify the likely single overriding problem to which most of the problems in the department may be owing.

T/P-11-03

Topic Emphasis:	Methods Improvement
Additional Topics:	Change Management, Decision Making, Motivation

---

The Lab Team

You are supervisor of the hospital's laboratory. Some of your employees work in teams, and their output is recorded on a team basis. In one of the teams Mary, Bob, and Jim work together. Each of them works at one station for an hour and then exchange, so all three employees perform each of the three tests at different times. The three employees decided themselves to operate this way, and you have never objected to the plan.

Lately, however, the hospital systems engineer has been studying conditions in your department. He timed Mary, Bob, and Jim on each of the tests and recorded the following information:

Time Per Test (In Minutes)

	Test #1	*Test #2*	*Test #3*	*Total*
Mary	3	4	4½	11½
Bob	3½	3½	3	10
Jim	5	3½	4½	13
				34½

The engineer observed that with the employees rotating, the average time for all three tests was one-third of the total time, or 11 1/2 minutes per complete three-test cycle. If, however, Mary worked in the number-one spot, Jim in the number-two spot, and Bob in the number-three spot, the total time would be 9 1/2 minutes—a reduction of more than 17 percent. Such a reduction in time would amount to a saving of more than 80 minutes each day. In other words, the output lost is about the same as that which would occur if the three employees loafed for a total of 80 minutes in an eight-hour day. If this time were used for more productive effort, output would be increased by more than 20 percent.

The systems engineer submitted a report to you, with a copy to your boss, recommending that you give Mary, Bob, and Jim the fixed assignments that would increase their output more than 20 percent.

Questions

1. What do you stand to gain by immediately giving the three employees the recommended fixed assignments?
2. What might you *lose* by mandating the new assignments?
3. Under what circumstances might you feel compelled to make the recommended assignments?
4. Could there be any circumstances under which you might wish to leave things as they are? What might these circumstances be?
5. By what other means could you improve team productivity?

GROUP 4

Primary Focus: TASK
Secondary Focus: SELF

T/S-01-01 (E)

Topic Emphasis: Change Management
Additional Topics: Methods Improvement, Personal Effectiveness

---

Changes in Office Practice

This exercise encourages you to consider changes in office practice which have occurred during the time you have been working. Under each of the headings given below, list as many items as you can think of which are now accepted as parts of your office activities but which, when you began working however many years ago, were either not in existence or not employed where you worked. These items may be either equipment you now have but did not have then, or techniques or practices which are now employed but which were not previously used.

After naming each item note approximately how many years you have been familiar with its use and indicate, if pertinent, what you did before things were done this way. Also, consider how well you believe you did— or did not—adapt to each such change with which you were faced.

1. Written communication—preparation of originals.
2. Written communication—preparation of copies.
3. Correspondence transmittal.
4. Financial transaction preparation and recording.
5. Verbal message transmission.
6. Record storage and retrieval.
7. Other changes in how you were required to do business.

T/S-06-01

Topic Emphasis:	General Management Practice
Additional Topics:	Communication, Leadership, Personal Effectiveness

---

A Tough Day for Lydia Michaels

Lydia Michaels was appointed to the newly created position of assistant director of nursing service at James Memorial, a general hospital serving a rapidly expanding suburban community. James Memorial is in the midst of a building program which will add 70 beds to the present 92 beds. Michaels, a registered nurse with nine years' experience, most recently served as day supervisor. She became assistant director when the first 25 of the additional 70 beds were within 60 days of opening, and it became her task to determine the staffing requirements for these first new beds and ultimately for the remainder of the new beds.

Michaels developed a master staffing plan based on providing each unit with a core staff set at 90 percent of the staff required at average expected census. To compensate for instances of understaffing she created a float pool to augment staff as needed.

One Tuesday morning James Memorial Hospital received word that local flash flooding was a possibility and that they should be prepared for flood-related activity. About the same time Michaels learned that one of her key people, the head nurse of the largest medical/surgical unit, had become seriously ill during the night.

From her float pool, already depleted by vacations and illness, Michaels was able to pull one practical nurse with emergency room experience. She then located two staff nurses with similar experience and told them they might be called to the emergency room and that if this happened they could expect to be asked to stay after the regular shift. She then made arrangements to cover their regular positions with float personnel should the move be necessary.

As for the large unit without its regular head nurse, Michaels was tempted to step into the breach herself since she had run the unit for two years and knew it well. However, she had no idea how long this coverage would be necessary, and she did not want to spread herself too thin by assuming an additional burden when she may be needed elsewhere. After brief consideration she decided to place the unit under the temporary direction of an energetic young staff nurse, Miss Carson. She had been aware of Carson's work for a number of weeks and had in fact considered using her in a charge capacity in the near future.

Local flood waters rose, boosted by heavy rain which also triggered a rash of traffic accidents. Emergency room activity stepped up considerably, and it became necessary to make the changes she had provided for.

That day, in a seven-hour span, the emergency room handled as many visits as in a peak 24-hour day and did so with patient waiting time no longer than usual. Asked later if the hospital's disaster plan (a number of elements of which had been put into effect) appeared adequate, Michaels was able to suggest that some procedures be strengthened in specific ways.

Instructions

In the case description there are numerous examples of the basic management functions: *planning, organizing, directing, coordinating,* and *controlling*. Identify as many of these instances as possible. (Note that many times a single activity will include elements of two or more of the basic functions in combination. However, on close examination one function will usually be found to be dominant.)

T/S-06-02

Topic Emphasis: General Management Practice
Additional Topics: Communication, People Problems,
                        Personal Effectiveness

The Fates Versus Harvey Brown

Harvey Brown, accounting supervisor at James Memorial Hospital, had every reason to feel that this had been "one of *those* days." Feeling more like Charlie Brown the perennial loser than Harvey Brown the accountant, he recounted the highlights of his Monday (did it always have to be *Monday*?):

- At 7:30 A.M. his car refused to start. He had to call a fellow employee for a ride, then call and arrange for his car to be towed and repaired.
- Abigail called in sick, and with Susan on vacation he had insufficient help in the department. A report which had to be finished that day lay partially completed beside Abigail's typewriter. After considerable asking around, he was able to borrow some typing time to complete the report.
- He received word that there would probably be an unanticipated general pay increase for hourly rated employees. This meant he would have to revise the manpower portion of the just-completed budget for the coming fiscal year.
- He lost the button off his shirt collar.
- He discovered there were some errors in the column totals on a spread sheet he had to use that day. Since Abigail had done the addition and he could find no one else to take care of it, he set about correcting it himself. He had hardly started when his calculator jammed. He was unable to clear it, so he put in a call for a service representative and did the work on one of the other machines in the office.
- Just before noon he learned that his car was ready. The price was staggering, and they could not deliver it. He arranged for a friend to take him to the garage at lunch time.
- The administrator's 1:00 P.M. staff meeting went longer than the usual one hour. Seeing that this was going to happen, Harvey excused himself long enough to call personnel and ask them if the job applicant he was to interview at 2:00 P.M. would be kind enough to remain an extra half hour.
- After an unsatisfactory interview he asked personnel to find him some more applicants for the open position.
- He returned to his office to find two of his employees arguing loudly over who was responsible for a task which had recently been created. He listened to both parties, sent one on an errand to provide some cooling-off time, and made himself a note to have one job description revised.

- He postponed a performance evaluation he had planned to conduct that afternoon because it involved one of the two arguing employees.
- His right shoelace broke.
- Through follow-up, he discovered that an employee had not yet provided the necessary information for the completion of the uniform financial report. Resisting the temptation to stay late and do the work himself, he spoke with the delinquent employee and stressed that he expected the information no later than noon the following day.
- Based on requests received in response to an earlier memo, he developed a vacation schedule for his department for the coming six months.
- He left the hospital one hour later than his usual quitting time, relieved that Monday had come to an end.

Instructions

Most of the foregoing items involve performance of one or more of the basic management functions: *planning, organizing, directing, coordinating,* and *controlling.* For each appropriate item, identify that management function or functions most descriptive of Harvey Brown's activity. (In some instances you may recognize two or three such functions; however, you will usually be able to recognize *one* function as dominant.)

T/S-06-03

> *Topic Emphasis:*   General Management Practice
> *Additional Topics:*   Communication, People Problems, Personal Effectiveness

---

Sharon's Day

Sharon Smith is secretary to the administrator of County General Hospital. Last year County General merged administratively with the neighboring Rehabilitation Center, and at about the same time opened its own long-term care facility. The administrator of County General was elevated to the position of executive director of the entire complex. Sharon was promoted to a secretarial job of considerably increased scope. As well as serving as secretary to the executive director, she was also made responsible for the supervision of the central administrative office staff.

One Thursday in May when Sharon came to work the first thing she did was make several telephone calls concerned with arranging banquet facilities for a retirement dinner. She had just made tentative arrangements subject to the approval of the executive director when she received a call advising her that one of the clerks in the duplicating room had reported sick. This concerned her because she was aware of a large printing job that had to be completed that day. Since the printing may or may not be accomplished with one less person present, she alerted the department to check with her periodically to see if assistance was needed in collating and bundling printed material.

At about mid-morning, Sharon finalized travel arrangements for the executive director to attend a conference in Chicago and typed a brief schedule and list of travel connections for him.

Shortly before lunch the administrative office receptionist reported that her typewriter was making strange noises and that the carriage refused to return correctly. After briefly examining the machine, Sharon put in a call to the local service representative. She made note of the time she did so and the time he promised to arrive.

After lunch she spent an hour researching journal articles dealing with a topic the executive director had selected for a speech. Interspersed with this activity, she also: called the office machine service and reminded them that the appointed time had arrived and their service representative was not there yet; delayed the office messenger's first afternoon round for 30 minutes so the messenger could help with collating duties; gave a clerical employee an interpretation of hospital policy regarding vacations; and reminded the executive director that he had an appointment across town in one hour and should allow himself 30 minutes' travel time.

Near the end of the afternoon she called the person who had reported sick to determine if she would be in the following day. Told that the employee would probably be there, Sharon then made several brief notes concerning items which she felt should be handled during the first half of the following day.

Instructions

In the foregoing brief description of one day's activities, identify as many of the basic management functions—*planning, organizing, directing, coordinating,* and *controlling*—as you can find. Keep in mind the possibility that more than one function may be present at the same time in the same activity, and that in numerous instances the performance of one function triggers the necessity for the performance of another.

GROUP 5

Primary Focus: SELF
Secondary Focus: PEOPLE

S/P-05-01

Topic Emphasis: Delegation
Additional Topics: Communication, Motivation,
Personal Effectiveness

"If You Want Things Done Well . . ."

John Miller, manager of laundry and linen for City Medical Center, dreaded the one day he had to spend each month doing the statistical report for his department. Miller was responsible for all laundry and linen activities in the 800-bed hospital, two smaller satellite facilities, and several municipal agencies whose linen needs the hospital filled. At one time the report had been relatively simple, but as Miller's scope of responsibility grew and administration requested increasingly more detailed information the report had become more complicated. Miller had simply modified his method of preparing the report each time a new requirement was placed upon him, so there was no written procedure for the report's preparation.

Faced once again with the time-consuming report—and confronted, as usual, with several problems demanding his immediate attention—John Miller decided it was time to delegate the preparation of the report to his assistant, Bill Curtis. He called Curtis to his office, gave him a copy of the previous month's report and a set of forms, and said, "I'm sure you've seen this. I want you to take care of it from now on. I've been doing it for a long time, but it's getting to be a real pain and I've got more important things to do than to allow myself to be tied up with routine clerical work."

Curtis spent perhaps half a minute skimming the report before he said, "I'm sure I can do it if I start on the right foot. How about walking me through it—doing one with me so I can get the hang of it?"

Miller said, "Look, my objective in giving you this is to save me some time. If I have to hold your hand I may as well do it myself." He grinned as he added, "Besides, if I can do it then anyone with half a brain ought to be able to do it."

Without further comment Curtis left the office with the report and the forms. Miller went to work on other matters.

Later that day Curtis stopped Miller in the corridor—they met while going in opposite directions—and said, "John, I'm glad I caught you. I've got three or four questions about the report, mostly concerning how you come up with the count and the percentages for the satellites." He started to pull a folded sheet of paper out of his back pocket.

Miller barely slowed. "Sorry, Bill, but I can't take the time. I'm on my way to a meeting." As he hurried past Curtis he called out over his shoulder, "You'll just have to puzzle it out for yourself. After all, I had to do the same thing."

The following day when the report was due, Miller found Curtis's work on his desk when he returned from lunch. He flipped through it to assure himself that all the blanks had been filled in, then he scrawled his signature in the usual place. However, something caught his eye—a number which appeared to be far out of line with anything he had encountered in previous reports. He took out two earlier reports and began a line-by-line comparison. He quickly discovered that Curtis had made a crucial error near the beginning and had carried this mistake through successive calculations.

Miller was angry with Curtis. The day was more than half gone and he would have to drop everything else and spend the rest of the afternoon reworking the figures so the report could be submitted on time.

Miller was still working at 4:30 P.M. when Pete Anderson, the engineering manager, appeared in the doorway and said, "I thought we were going to rework your preventive maintenance schedule this afternoon. What are you up to, anyway?"

Miller threw down his pencil and snapped, "I'm proving an old saying."

"Meaning what?"

"Meaning—if you want something done right, do it yourself."

Instructions

1. Miller committed several significant errors in "delegating" the statistical report to Curtis. Identify at least three such errors in the case description.
2. Using as many steps as you believe necessary, describe how this instance of delegation might have been accomplished properly.

S/P-14-01

Topic Emphasis: Personal Effectiveness
Additional Topics: Communication, Leadership

One of the Gang

You have been employed in the hospital's business office for nearly 11 years. You began in a clerical capacity and have worked your way up through several of the jobs in the department. You consider yourself friends with all 14 other business office employees, and at least 2 of them you number among your closest friends.

Recently you were appointed business office manager. You wanted the position, and you willingly accepted it. You believe that although one or two persons within the department may feel some slight resentment over your appointment they are, for the most part, supportive. However, you realize that as a supervisor it may sometimes be necessary for you to do things which are not consistent with your feelings for this group of people with whom you have worked for so long.

Questions

1. Should you find it necessary to "pull away" to any extent from those people with whom you have worked for so long?
2. How do you believe you should go about reestablishing a long-term relationship with your former coworkers?

GROUP 6

Primary Focus: SELF
Secondary Focus: TASK

S/T-05-01

Topic Emphasis: Delegation
Additional Topics: General Management Practice,
Leadership, Personal Effectiveness

Take Your Choice

You are a registered nurse with 20 years' experience, and you have spent 10 years as nursing director in a 65-bed rural hospital. You recently applied for the position of assistant director of nursing at a 375-bed city hospital. During your initial interview the director of nursing posed four sets of "conditions" and asked you to state which of these best described the circumstances under which you believed such a position should be taken. The "conditions" are:

a. You step into the job with the full authority and responsibility of the position as experienced by your predecessor.
b. You assume the full authority of the position but have somewhat reduced responsibility because of your newness to the job.
c. You have equal responsibility and authority but at a lesser level than your predecessor, leaving you room to "grow" in the position.
d. You assume the full responsibility of the position but can exercise less authority than your predecessor (again, because you are "new").

Questions

1. Describe the advantages and disadvantages of each set of "conditions" relative to (a) yourself and (b) the institution.
2. Under which set of "conditions" should you consider taking the job? Why?

S/T-14-01

Topic Emphasis:	Personal Effectiveness
Additional Topics:	Change Management,
	Communication, Time Management

How Can You Possibly
Schedule under These Conditions?

The maintenance department of General Hospital consisted of George Wilson, a working supervisor, and three other employees. These four men took care of all mechanical and electrical equipment with the exception of biomedical equipment. They also did limited remodeling, painting, and building repairs.

As a matter of practice all maintenance services were supposed to be rendered as needed. However, when something needed fixing, painting, or changing, Wilson and his workers would do it "when they could get to it." Although all four men appeared to be working all the time they seemed never to be caught up. There were numerous complaints about delays in obtaining service.

Wilson's department head, the director of building services, urged him to put all of the institution's equipment on a preventive maintenance schedule and to schedule all other jobs that came to the maintenance crew. Wilson resisted on the grounds that too many maintenance activities did not lend themselves to prediction or scheduling. Besides, he reasoned, the development of the schedule would simply represent more time spent nonproductively. However, the director was insistent, and reluctantly Wilson set about creating a one-month schedule for his group.

In developing his schedule, Wilson looked at all available working days for the month for all maintenance personnel. He scheduled his three employees at 100 percent, dedicating half their time to preventive maintenance and the other half to known painting and remodeling projects. Of his own time he scheduled 75 percent on preventive maintenance, leaving the balance open for supervision and coordination.

The first day the new schedule went into effect an air conditioner failure caused Wilson to alter the schedule. The air conditioner repair carried over into the second day, and on the third day the mechanism of an automatic door jammed in an open position. By the end of the first week Wilson's desk was piled high with maintenance service requests for small repair jobs. So it went for the entire month.

At the end of one month, Wilson submitted a brief report to the director of building services saying he was forced to abandon the practice of scheduling maintenance. The department's work, he again reasoned, was sufficiently variable and unpredictable to make any kind of scheduling impractical if not impossible.

Instructions

1. Identify the weaknesses in Wilson's approach to scheduling that essentially guaranteed failure before he began.
2. Describe how Wilson might go about compensating for the shortcomings that caused the failure of his scheduling system.

S/T-14-02

Topic Emphasis: Personal Effectiveness
Additional Topics: Change Management, Decision
Making, Leadership

Where Do You Begin?

You have just taken over as director of nursing service. You came from another hospital, but you are familiar with this institution because you once worked here for two years (ending five years ago).

During your first week you are faced with:

- Meeting your assistant director, who clearly thinks she should have been made director;
- Complaints from a number of nurses who claim they never have weekends off;
- Clear cases of understaffing on evenings and nights;
- Overstaffing on the day shift in most units;
- A high percentage of part-time nurses who have been permitted to work "when available";
- Several staff physicians who are in the habit of giving narcotic orders orally or by telephone and writing them out "when I get the chance";
- Information suggesting that an outside organization is trying to get all of your registered nurses interested in a union.

Questions

1. Where do you begin the effort to "clean up" your department? What do you see as your first priority, and why?
2. Depending on your answer to the preceding question, what would you see as your second priority? Why?
3. How many of these problems are inextricably related to each other?

S/T-14-03

Topic Emphasis:	Personal Effectiveness
Additional Topics:	Communication, Time Management

"Where Does the Time Go?"

Kay Thatcher, director of staff education, decided she had to get organized. Recently her work days had been running well beyond quitting time, cutting noticeably into the time required by her family responsibilities, but instead of going down, her backlog of work was growing.

Inspired by an article she read about planning and setting priorities, Kay decided to try planning each day's activities at the end of the previous day. This Monday Kay came to the office with her day planned out to the last minute. During the morning she had to complete a report on a recent learning-needs analysis, write the performance appraisals of two part-time instructors, and assemble the balance of the materials for a two-hour class she was scheduled to conduct that afternoon. After lunch she had to conduct the class, complete the schedule of the next three months' training activities (now ten days overdue), and prepare notices—which should be posted this very day—for two upcoming classes.

Kay got off to a good start; she finished the report before 10:00 and turned her attention to the performance evaluations. However, at that time the interruptions began. In the next two hours she was interrupted six times—three telephone calls and three visitors. The calls were all business calls. Two of the visitors had legitimate problems, one of them taking perhaps a half-hour to resolve. The other visitor was a fellow supervisor simply passing the time of day. Neither performance evaluation was completed, and the training materials were assembled in time only because Kay put them together during lunch while juggling a sandwich at her desk.

Kay's afternoon class ran 20 minutes overtime because of legitimate questions and discussion. When she returned to her office she discovered she had a visitor, a good-humored, talkative salesman from whom Kay occasionally bought audiovisual materials. He "happened to be in the area and just dropped in." He stayed for an hour and a half.

After the salesman left, Kay spent several minutes simply wondering what to do next. The performance appraisals, the three-month schedule, the class notices—all were overdue. Deciding on the class notices because they were the briefest task before her, she dashed off both notices in longhand and asked the nursing department secretary to type them, run them off, and post them immediately. She then tackled the training schedule.

When Kay again looked up from her work it was nearly an hour past quitting time. She still had a long way to go on the schedule and had not yet gotten started on the two performance appraisals. As she swept her work aside for the day she sadly reflected that she had not accomplished two-thirds of what she intended to do that day in spite of all her planning. She decided, however, to try again; when she could get a few minutes of quiet time late in the evening, she would plan her next day's activity.

On her way out of the hospital she happened to glance at the main bulletin board. The small satisfaction she felt when she saw the posted class notices vanished instantly when she discovered that both were incorrect—the dates and times of the two classes had been interchanged.

Questions

1. What errors did Kay commit in her approach to planning and the establishment of priorities?
2. In what respects could Kay have improved her use of time on the "blue Monday" described in the case?

S/T-14-04

> *Topic Emphasis:* Personal Effectiveness
> *Additional Topics:* Communication, Time Management

The Salesman

As the door closed behind her departing visitor Janet Mills, the central supply supervisor, glumly reflected that she had just lost an hour which she could ill afford to lose. She would either have to forgo completing the schedule she was working on or be late for an upcoming meeting.

The hour had been lost because of a visit from a pleasant but marginally aggressive salesman trying to acquaint her with the "greatest little thing ever to come along." Janet, as was her practice, consented to see him although she resented the intrusion.

This incident, occurring on a Friday, made Janet realize that she had lost time to four such drop-in visits this week alone. She did not like the idea of simply saying no or otherwise trying to avoid people who wanted to see her, but she was becoming more aware that her work was beginning to suffer because of such demands on her time.

Instruction

Develop some guidelines which might help Janet and other supervisors deal with the problem of drop-in visitors.

Chapter 6

"The Threat": A Major Case in Interpersonal Relations

THE SETTING

County General Medical Center is a large, multi-institutional health facility. It is headed by a president. Reporting to the president are four persons, each bearing the title of director of one of the institutions. We are interested in an occurrence within the largest of the components, the 1,000-bed, acute-care County Hospital.

County Hospital is the original institution around which the center was built. The hospital was in a constant state of either expansion or planning for expansion until only recently. However, current long-range planning suggests that the period of rapid expansion may have come to an end.

THE PEOPLE

Ronald Davis, 37, is director of County Hospital. He has been there four years, the first two as assistant director for patient services. He holds master's degrees in both hospital administration and finance. His total work experience is in health care, and all of it has been in hospital operations. He is respected in the field and is an energetic, dynamic individual known to take a great deal of enjoyment from his work. He is on the premises six and sometimes seven days a week. His workday customarily starts before 7:00 A.M. and often runs 12 to 14 hours. He is respected by his management team and by many individual employees, most of whom he knows by name. It is widely thought that Davis will be the next president of the center when the current president retires in two years.

Ralph Grant, 34, is assistant director for personnel services. His total experience in health care consists of the two years he has been at the hospital. He is considered a highly knowledgeable specialist in labor relations, and Davis recruited him to deal specifically with a major union organizing attempt. Grant is credited with being the moving force in reversing an unfavorable trend in employee relations and with keeping the hospital nonunion.

Grant is highly respected for his knowledge of labor relations and for his bargaining and negotiating skills. However, upon prolonged exposure the more-than-casual observer can pick up noticeable undercurrents of distrust, if not fear, of Grant on the part of some employees. Opinions have quietly circulated among employees that during the union organization drive Grant employed techniques which were unethical, if not illegal.

Carl Miller, 36, is assistant director for support services. Among the departments reporting to him are housekeeping, food services, engineering and maintenance, and systems engineering. Miller has been with County Hospital slightly more than six months, having come from local industry. He holds an undergraduate degree in general business and a master's degree in industrial management. He does not impress people as a dynamic individual, but he has been reasonably successful in leading the managers who report to him. He is generally well liked.

NOTE: The persons described so far are part of a relatively young management group. County Hospital has a history of rapid turnover in management positions. This turnover peaked in the early months of Davis's administration and seems to have leveled off since then. However, among some of the older employees these members of management are derisively referred to as "the young Turks" and are frequently the subject of comments concerning the bringing of "industrial methods" into the hospital. Generally overlooked in these comments is the continued enhancement of County Hospital's reputation for quality care plus the fact that in this most recent year, for the first time in more than a decade, County Hospital did not operate at a deficit.

Walter Sutton, 49, is a manager of a five-employee department known as systems engineering. He reports to Carl Miller. Sutton, originally a school teacher, has spent 24 years with County Hospital. He began as employment manager and later became an administrative assistant. When the hospital first became interested in data processing, Sutton, through part-time study, became a computer programmer and later a systems analyst. As the function grew to include other activities such as industrial engineering, other persons were added and Sutton grew into a position as manager of a small group.

In addition to Sutton, the department includes three systems analysts who are best described as management engineers, one mathematician who operates as a staff specialist in operations research, and one planner. For the four months prior to the time Miller was hired, Sutton had looked after the activities of assistant director for support services on an acting basis.

Edward Barnes, 52, is a systems analyst reporting to Sutton. He has been with County Hospital for six years. His background is equally divided between industrial engineering in industry and in the hospital setting. He is generally regarded as a competent systems analyst, but also as something of a loner who does not take direction well and who prefers to pursue lengthy in-depth projects on which he can work alone. Although coming across as somewhat surly, he was nevertheless sufficiently popular to be elected president of the Employees' Activity Guild.

THE SITUATION

One Monday morning Carl Miller arrived at his office at his customary 8:00 A.M., thirty minutes before normal starting time. The first person he met was his secretary, Mae, who told him Walt Sutton had mentioned to her on the way out Friday that he would like some time with Miller Monday morning on a matter of importance.

Thinking back over the past week to some comments by Sutton, Miller wondered if it had something to do with Ed Barnes who was due for a semiannual performance evaluation. On at least three recent occasions Sutton had mentioned that he felt Barnes was getting increasingly difficult to manage, and that Barnes was giving him a particularly hard time about staying on an expensive but apparently nonproductive study which Barnes wanted to continue. Sutton had expressed some apprehension about the performance review he was to discuss with Barnes on Monday. He thought he had let things go long enough, and felt it was about time Barnes was advised of who was running the group and calling the shots.

Miller knew that Barnes and Sutton had never been fond of each other, but he was unaware of any particular antagonism between the two. Miller told Mae to go ahead and tell Sutton he would see him right away, but Mae had no sooner left to do so when Davis summoned Miller to discuss a management problem of some urgency. The matter consumed half the morning.

When Miller returned to his office he found several message slips on his desk, two of which were checked "urgent." With them was a note from

Mae that read: "Walt was looking for you again. He said he would see you at lunch if you can't get back to him before then."

What had shaped up as a hectic morning soon became a hectic day. As Miller was reaching to buzz his secretary, he received a visit from Arthur Morrison, manager of engineering and maintenance. Morrison was accompanied by the supervisor of an outside construction crew. Several problems had to be worked out immediately so the waiting crew could resume work.

Once during his meeting Miller caught a glimpse of Sutton through his office door. Sutton had ducked out of the larger office where his department was located and looked in through the glass. Sutton caught Miller's eyes and raised his eyebrows in question. Miller returned with a brief nod and a small hand signal which he hoped would say that he would get with him as soon as possible. However, just before noon when Miller was concluding the business with his visitors, he received a call from personnel. The employment manager, on Ralph Grant's instructions, had made a luncheon interview appointment for Miller to talk with a likely candidate for a management position in food service. Miller started for the personnel office. He went by way of Sutton's office to see if he could catch him for a moment, but Sutton was not there.

Miller kept his luncheon appointment. It was a productive interview but consumed two hours of his day. When he returned to his office at 2:00 P.M. he found two visitors from outside the hospital waiting for him, again accompanied by Morrison. They were from a local environmental protection organization and had called because the hospital was past the deadline date for submitting a refuse-disposal plan which would permit them to eliminate incineration. Morrison was to have developed and submitted the plan for Miller's approval. This had not been done, and Miller only now realized that he had put off the follow-up which he ordinarily pursued in such matters.

Shortly after he had begun dealing with his visitors, Carl Miller noticed Ed Barnes in the hall outside his office. Barnes had repeated Sutton's earlier move, stepping out of the larger office to see if Miller was available, and backing off when he saw the visitors. Miller thought that with Sutton and now Barnes attempting to see him perhaps the two were squabbling. He decided he had better talk with them both at the earliest opportunity.

The meeting with the pollution-control people was extremely difficult and dragged on for more than two hours. During that time Barnes and Sutton each appeared briefly in the hall at least three times. Just before 4:00 the two burst through the door of the larger office simultaneously. Sutton turned to his right and moved rapidly out of sight. Barnes turned left and looked into Miller's office. Before Barnes turned away, Miller caught a glimpse of red face and angry eyes.

It was about 4:15 when Miller got rid of his visitors. He immediately buzzed for his secretary and sent for Sutton who arrived in a matter of seconds appearing pale and obviously agitated.

"What's the trouble, Walt?" Miller asked.

"I just fired Barnes," Sutton said. "Something I should have done long ago. I told him to pack up and get the hell out of here. Now."

Miller said, "Cool down, Walt. I don't think you can do that. You remember what Davis says about this."

"I don't care what Davis says about this," Sutton yelled. "Barnes threatened to kill me. That guy is not working for me or this hospital, and you'd better back me up if you're any kind of boss."

"Hold on a minute. Temper isn't going to get us anywhere. Just try to give me a straight story about what happened."

"Not much of anything happened except that I gave him a lousy performance review—I told you I was going to do that, and I tried to get to you to let you see it first. He didn't like it. He got mad and got mouthy, and one thing led to another and he threatened to kill me. So I fired him."

"Okay, Walt. I'd like you to do two things. Go tell Ed I want to see him for a minute. Then get that performance review; we're going to need it."

Sutton left, and less than a minute later Barnes was sitting across the desk from Carl Miller. Before Miller could speak, Barnes calmly asked, "Sutton told you he fired me?"

"Yes," Miller answered.

"And he told you he gave me a bad performance evaluation?"

"Yes, though I haven't seen it yet and don't know how bad it is."

"It's bad, believe me. It's the poorest I've ever seen. I don't know how a boss can give me good reviews for years, and then suddenly I'm lousy on all counts. I doesn't figure."

Barnes's eyes narrowed, and he glared across the desk at Miller. His words were quiet but coldly uttered. He said, "That evaluation is a smear. An out-and-out lying, underhanded smear, and I'm telling you, mister whiz-kid boss, that if you and your flunky Sutton do this to me you'll hear from me through a lawyer and you'll pay for it. I have a good reputation in my field and in this town, and I'm not going to have it ruined by a boss who doesn't have the brains to do his job and a Johnny-come-lately manager who doesn't know the score."

At that moment Sutton reappeared at the office door. He held up a pink sheet of paper—the performance evaluation. Miller waved him into the office and glanced briefly at the evaluation. As Barnes had contended, it was bad. Every item on it except punctuality was rated at the lower end of the scale. Looking from the paper to the men Miller sensed that the two were going to begin speaking at once. He held up his hand to forestall them while he dialed Ralph Grant's extension. Miller was told that Grant was busy with a visitor; he asked the secretary to interrupt. Once on the telephone Miller said only, "Ralph, I have a personnel problem that can't wait. It involves a hasty firing, and I have a couple of angry people with me right now. We need to see you."

Miller took the performance evaluation, and he and Sutton and Barnes went to Ralph Grant's office. Grant had excused his visitor. They all took seats, and Grant closed the door. It was approximately 4:30 P.M.

Grant's eyes quickly swept over the three faces. He settled on Miller and asked, "What's the story?"

Miller handed over the performance evaluation and said, "Apparently Walt, here, reviewed Ed today. Routine performance evaluation, but indicating lots of problems. The review is less than satisfactory. Isn't that right, Walt?"

"A lot less than satisfactory," snapped Sutton. Barnes muttered an obscenity.

Grant turned to Barnes and said, "Talk to us, not to yourself, and say things that mean something. Is that right? He gave you a bad review?"

"A rotten review. He's had it in for me for months. Don't ask me why, but it seems I haven't been able to do anything to please this guy."

Grant turned to Sutton and asked, "Is that right?"

"His performance was way below satisfactory in my estimation," Sutton said. "It never has been acceptable to me, and I've finally had it. It's about time he knows who runs the department. I have no use for one guy who piddles along at his own pace on the things he wants to do, won't take direction, and won't account for results. I've watched him grow more and more independent, and I've watched his work go from bad to worse. I'm not putting up with it any longer."

"You fired him?", Grant asked.

"Yes, I fired him," Sutton said, his anger rising. "I couldn't even discuss the review with him. He doesn't take criticism at all. With every point I tried to go over, he called me names. References to my size, that's his favorite thing—a cut-rate Napoleon, he called me. He said I was incompetent, that I wasn't fit to manage, and he called me just about every foul thing under the sun and I got mad and I fired him. And he should stay fired."

Grant turned to Barnes and asked. "Did you say those things?"

Barnes shrugged and said, "Guess I did. In so many words, more or less. He made me mad. It would make you mad, too, to get an unfair raking-over like that."

"And he threatened to kill me," Sutton said.

Grant asked, "Before or after you fired him?"

"After. He got up close to me, waving his finger under my nose and talking practically through his teeth. He said something like, 'Don't you think you can do this to me and not pay and pay heavy. I know where you live, I know what your wife looks like, I know the places you go, and I know the things you do. And if you fire me, the first time I see you outside of here you're a dead man.'"

Grant made a couple of notes on a pad. He turned to Barnes and asked, "Did you say that?"

Again Barnes shrugged and said, "More or less."

Grant said, "Go home, Ed, and stay there tomorrow until I call you. Sometime tomorrow afternoon I'd like to talk to you about this. We'll sort it all out then. I can't give you any answers right now."

After Barnes left Grant turned his attention to Sutton and said, "Walt, you know Davis had made it a blanket rule that nobody gets fired without his approval."

"I know," Sutton said defensively. "But this was different. There was no time for his approval."

"Look," Grant said, "His say-so is precisely what there should have been time for. He's said time and time again he wants no one fired in anger, ever. It's necessary to clear it with him to give you a cooling-off period if nothing else. This action of yours is completely contrary to one of the director's most strongly stated policies."

Grant turned to Miller and asked, "What's your impression of Barnes?"

"I don't know him that well. I imagine I know him the least of all the people who work in my departments. Ordinarily he's quiet. A couple of people have had minor things to say about his unpleasant manner on occasion, but there's really nothing I know beyond that."

Grant said to Sutton, "Walt, come in tomorrow at the usual time. I don't know if the firing is going to stand. I doubt that it will." Sutton's eyebrows shot up, and his angry look returned.

Grant held up a hand and said, "Walt, I know how you feel. So far Davis has never failed to back up a manager on a firing if there was reason behind it and it was cleared with him. This is different, or at least it may be different. We'll just have to see. Now please try to simmer down. Go home. We'll talk with you in the morning."

Sutton left. Grant sighed wearily and said, "Carl, my boy, you dug up a good one this time." He reached for the telephone and dialed Davis.

Before going to Davis's office Grant took a few minutes to check some records having to do with performance evaluations. In particular, he checked Sutton's prior reviews of Barnes.

"This is interesting," Grant observed. "In one way Barnes is quite right. There are several reviews here on which he was satisfactory right down the line. Some even have a few above-average ratings here and there. It's got to be puzzling for Barnes to hear Sutton saying he's never been happy with him since he's always rated him acceptable. On the other hand, when you look at the statistics on the evaluations done by all of our managers you discover that Sutton is a high rater. Looking at all the ones he's done, and looking at the tabulations of these ratings, it appears that to Sutton 'average' performance is somewhere between 'above average' and 'superior.' He seems to operate like he's actually down-rating by giving out something less than an outstanding review.''

On the way to Davis's office Grant said to Miller, ''You've got quite a problem on your hands, and you're going to have to take a hand in deciding what to do.''

Instructions

Thoroughly analyze the incident and all occurrences leading to it. Prepare yourself to explain:

1. what factors you believe permitted the incident to occur; and
2. what you believe could be done to correct the resulting situation.

Your explanation would appropriately include your impressions of the organization, the philosophy of operating management, and the apparent right or wrong of any applicable hospital policies.

It is suggested that you carefully consider the conduct of the five principals—Davis, Grant, Miller, Sutton, and Barnes—and decide which of their actions may have been right and which may have been wrong, and why you believe them to be right or wrong.

In brief, you should be attempting to cut through a tangle of errors to determine what happened, why it happened, and what should be done about it.

AND HAVING DONE SO

The foregoing tale was presented as an *open-ended case*, that is, one that takes you just so far, leaving you to decide on a solution or possible solutions. A *closed-ended case* is one for which you are given an ending, that is, you not only know what happened, but you also know what corrective action was taken. Consider the following ''ending'' for ''The Threat.''

"THE THREAT": CONTINUED

On the way to Davis's office Grant said to Miller, "You've got quite a problem on your hands, and you're going to have to take a hand in deciding what to do. Chances are we're going to overturn the firing. This will destroy both you and Sutton as managers with Barnes, and it could weaken you both with a large part of the organization. You should take advantage of this to do some housecleaning and organizational rearranging. My observations suggest—and these are observations and impressions only—that your man Sutton is a loyal, conscientious employee, but he doesn't know how to manage. He never has and probably never will. His employee, Barnes, is said to be generally unpleasant, might be relatively unproductive, and doesn't take supervision well. Also, he's thin-skinned and quick-tempered."

Miller remained with Grant and Davis for most of the evening discussing the situation and its implications. A course of action was put into effect at three meetings.

The first meeting was held the next day in one of the hospital's cafeterias. Present on instructions from the director were all members of the administrative staff and upper management, and as many individual managers and supervisors who were on the premises or who could be spared from their work.

Addressing the group Davis said, "I wanted to get with you as early as possible on a matter of some importance that has probably gone halfway around the hospital by this time, considering the ways news of this nature travels. Ed Barnes was fired yesterday afternoon. As director I have to perform an unpleasant first and overrule the manager who discharged Barnes and reinstate him subject to a limited form of disciplinary probation.

"I take this step in full appreciation of the impact it can have on the employees' view of a manager's authority, but I have to do this because the firing—and it may even have been deserved—was in direct contradiction of one of our most strongly stated policies. This rule exists so I can assure as well as possible that no one is ever discharged in anger. That's precisely what happened in this case. As a result of an angry exchange between two people, a man was fired. That cause for firing may really have existed is not the issue. The real issue is that an employee was discharged in anger, and in adherence to our policy I'm forced to reinstate that individual."

The second meeting was a brief session between Carl Miller and Edward Barnes late in the afternoon. The essence of Miller's communication with Barnes was: "The firing has been reversed and you've been reinstated.

Officially you're on strict 30-day disciplinary probation during which time your conduct is supposed to be carefully reviewed. Although your immediate supervisor acted contrary to policy and without authorization in firing you, he did so following strong provocation from you. You and your present supervisor will probably not be able to coexist in the same department. The probation is official, but on a less-than-official level I strongly suggest you make use of these 30 days to find another position. If you're cooperative in this matter and leave of your own accord, no one in another organization need know anything about what went on here these last couple of days. You'll be given the kind of reference ordinarily accorded the average satisfactory employee who leaves without prejudice. It is evident that you and Sutton are not able to get along with each other, and we feel you ought to have the opportunity to start over and establish a clean slate somewhere else. One of you had to leave, and we elected to retain Sutton, principally on the basis of length of service and potential future contributions."

The following morning Carl Miller met privately with Walter Sutton. The essence of this communication was: "Your actions in the arbitrary firing of Barnes and the subsequent reversal of that firing have pretty much destroyed any effectiveness you may have had as a manager. However, we recognize the contributions you have made to County Hospital over the years, and we sincerely believe you can continue contributing in areas of which you are knowledgeable. You are being relieved of your position as manager. Instead, you will function in the capacity of senior systems analyst in that department."

Sutton accepted the demotion with some initial resentment. However, within a few weeks he had adapted to his new role, and much later he confided to Miller that he had never really felt comfortable wearing the manager's hat and was rather glad he no longer had certain duties to worry about.

Approximately four weeks after the incident, Barnes gave notice of voluntary resignation. He had found another position and was returning to manufacturing.

Instructions

First, compare the results of your analysis of the open-ended version of the case with the "real" ending described in the closed-ended version. Chances are your possible solution does not strike you as being nearly as drastic as the "real" ending. If so, try to decide why things may have proceeded to such extremes.

Next, continue your analysis of the case to include the manner in which the problem was "solved." In your view, were the actions taken right? Wrong? And most importantly, do you believe this situation could have been handled better? If so, how?

(In dealing with the latter question, consider how matters had deteriorated before the problem came to higher management's attention. Most possible solutions will seem flawed in the sense that certain parties are either punished severely or escape punishment that may have been deserved. This should suggest that when a problem is permitted to develop to a point where damage has occurred, often nothing can be done to return things to their exact original order.)

Chapter 7

The In-Basket Exercise

A COMPREHENSIVE EXERCISE

The in-basket exercise is a comprehensive and effective simulation of many of the interrelated problems and conditions that a supervisor is likely to encounter. It can be structured to encompass virtually every element found in the day-to-day problem-solving and decision-making environment except one—the emotional involvement resulting from the knowledge that something is at stake. This, of course, is an element which remains forever absent from all situations except those that occur "for real." Except for the absence of real-world consequences, however, the in-basket exercise is an accurate representation of reality.

The in-basket exercise combines most features of case studies, role plays, and individual exercises into a single comprehensive exercise. The user of an in-basket exercise assumes the position of a character, much as in a role play, and from the viewpoint of that character deals with a series of questions, problems, telephone calls, and items of correspondence. In doing so the user pursues objectives related to:

- testing and sharpening skills used in problem solving and decision making;
- strengthening one's ability to organize problems as they arise, to "sort out" items as to importance and the likely required approach to solution;
- sharpening one's ability to establish priorities.

The in-basket exercise has a number of features that make it a valuable addition to any supervisory development activity. These features are:

1. It is as representative of reality as an exercise can be while still remaining an exercise. When properly structured and approached, it includes a realistic element of time pressure as well as a realistic mix of problems and situations.
2. It is a no-risk activity. Since it *is* an exercise, no harm is done if inappropriate responses are made.
3. When it is utilized within the context of an organized supervisory development activity, immediate feedback on one's responses is available.
4. Again as viewed within the context of an organized supervisory development program, the exercise produces attendee involvement. It is not possible for a participant to remain passive during an in-basket exercise.
5. Of the numerous supervisory skills which it addresses, the exercise especially encourages the development and refinement of delegation skills. Participants quickly recognize that one person cannot "do it all alone," and that some items should—and indeed must—be handled by others.
6. The exercise encourages participants to think of the organization as a whole, realizing that many things done in an organization have implications beyond one's own function or department.

FEATURES

The most effective in-basket exercises require the participants to "act" in roles one organizational level higher than their own positions. Even if you handle your own level's in-basket appropriately, handling your boss's in-basket will be a learning experience because it includes the challenge of territory you do not ordinarily cover. You are called upon to cope with the kinds of material your department head receives, material which will ordinarily include some of the kinds of problems you usually see *plus* additional situations you ordinarily would not handle.

One essential feature of an in-basket exercise is the element of time pressure. A reasonably tight time limit is set on the completion of the exercise. It is one thing to determine the disposition of a dozen or more in-basket items at your leisure; given an unlimited amount of time, most of us could do a high-quality job of it. However, it is another matter entirely to strive for quality results knowing that the clock may run out before the end is reached. Time pressure is an essential part of the in-basket exercise; few if any people in supervision can afford the luxury of dealing with their problems free of time considerations, so the time pressure becomes characteristic of the realism to be found in this form of exercise.

Within the in-basket exercise the participant must cope with a variety of problems, requests, correspondence, and telephone messages. Each item must be assessed for its importance and perhaps classified as to the kind of action required and the likely source of that action. For each item a decision must be made, a decision that either resolves the item or puts it in the proper framework for its eventual resolution.

In assessing the in-basket it is necessary to ask of each item:

1. What kind of problem is it? Is it truly mine, or my department's problem? Is it going to—or should it—involve other departments?
2. Is more information needed? If so, what kinds of information, and is it information I have available, or must I obtain it elsewhere?
3. How urgent is the situation? Must it be handled right now, or can it wait until later?
4. What is the scope of the problem? Can it be resolved in minutes, or will it require extended time and effort?

In making a decision or planning and ordering action in response to an in-basket item, you should also be responding to two basic questions:

1. Can—or should—this be dealt with right now or dealt with later?
2. Can—or should—I take care of this personally, or should it be delegated to someone?

USES

You may use the in-basket exercise to (a) evaluate your work habits and your approach to the job; and (b) practice your communications skills (since quick written responses are usually called for).

As a supervisory development activity the exercise may be used by itself or as part of a larger program. As part of a program, it is especially valuable in helping to vary the pace of the program and provide balance with other, less participative activities such as lectures and films. This exercise is particularly helpful in promoting an increased degree of participation from program attendees.

The in-basket exercise can also be a valuable opening exercise of a program. How the attendees fare and the questions and problems they raise as a result of the exercise can help determine the topics that should be covered in subsequent sessions.

DEVELOPING AN IN-BASKET EXERCISE

You can readily structure an in-basket exercise to serve any of several topic areas of importance to supervision. Foremost among generally pertinent topic areas are:

- *communication*—an exercise consisting mostly of items to which you must respond in writing within a limited time;
- *decision making*—a collection of problems, each of which requires a solution or a specific decision that could lead to a solution;
- *planning*—an exercise composed of items of varying degrees of urgency or importance which you must place in priority order;
- *delegation*—a number of items which must be taken care of by persons who work for you, with your emphasis on deciding *who* should take care of *what*.

An in-basket exercise may also be general in nature, involving a seemingly random array of items which cut across all of those mentioned in the foregoing list. Such an exercise, similar to the sample presented in this chapter, is suggested as the kind to use at the start of a supervisory development program. The feedback from an exercise of this nature can suggest the kinds of material to stress in other sessions.

In developing an in-basket exercise, first select the organizational position or *role* to be assumed by the user. Clearly define the organizational position of the role character relative to the remainder of that person's department. This is most easily done with a simple organization chart spelling out the names and positions of the role character's employees and, as necessary, the role character's manager and other persons in the organization.

Next, assemble a collection of representative messages—letters, memorandums, brief reports, telephone messages, notes, etc.—that would likely be encountered by the role character in a normal day's work. Include a variety of problems (unless you are structuring a single-purpose exercise) spread over a range of importance and urgency, a sampling of correspondence from inside as well as from outside the institution, and perhaps an item or two of an unusual nature. Also consider inserting one or two "interruptions" (refer to the sample exercise).

Where can you find material? Begin by looking in your own in-basket. Usually you can find several appropriate items in your own stack of correspondence and telephone messages; you might combine these with one or two short cases from Chapter 5 and invent a couple of items based on questions from Chapter 9.

When designing an exercise, establish the time it ought to require by going through it and timing yourself. Do not loaf along through the items; rather, give each the attention you would ordinarily give it if you knew you should really try to empty the basket before moving on to your next meeting, or whatever else may be on your schedule. If you are able to set a time in which you can just comfortably complete the exercise (remember, *you* assembled the exercise, so by knowing the items you have a head start on anyone else who may try it) chances are that it will offer a challenging element of time pressure to someone attempting the exercise. In any case, should the time you set prove to be inappropriate you can change it for subsequent uses of the exercise or you can add or delete items should you wish to preserve the time frame.

SAMPLE IN-BASKET EXERCISE:

Palmer's Friday

You are P. J. Palmer, assistant administrator of Wilton Community Hospital. You also "wear a second hat" in that you serve as the hospital's personnel director as well. You have occupied your present position for nearly four years.

Wilton Community Hospital is a 92-bed general hospital located in the village of Wilton, a semirural community of less than four thousand persons. The hospital is the community's second largest employer; the largest employer is Wilton Foods, a locally owned canning and food processing company.

Wilton Hospital is 28 miles from Center City. The hospital has a number of formal working agreements with Center City General Hospital to supply some service and support functions which Wilton, because of its size and the nature of its services, cannot adequately or economically provide. For instance, most of Wilton's nonroutine laboratory work is done at Center City General, and certain difficult cases are usually transferred to Center City General.

Wilton's pathology and radiology physicians' services are provided by groups that work out of Center City General. Wilton Hospital's anesthesiology, respiratory therapy, and physical therapy are provided on a contract basis by groups based in Center City.

Wilton Hospital has no laundry; it uses a hospital linen service located in Center City. Linen distribution and control is handled through the Wilton hospital's housekeeping department.

Staff has been relatively stable at Wilton Hospital, with significant turnover occurring in only one or two departments. Personnel have been readily available within the community except for registered nurses and licensed practical nurses. Like many hospitals in the state, Wilton Hospital has been unable to find nurses to fill all of its needs.

No employees of Wilton Community Hospital are unionized. However, there has been a great deal of union organizing activity among hospital employees in Center City.

With the exceptions of the hospital pharmacist and the medical records manager, the department heads who report to you are "up from the ranks" within Wilton Community Hospital. Since Wilton is not large relative to many other hospitals, your department heads are also first-line supervisors in that they directly supervise the nonmanagerial people who do the hands-on work.

The nine people who report directly to you are:

Sharon Kelly, secretary and personnel records clerk, is your secretary and the hospital's employee benefits coordinator and keeper of personnel records.

Jane Casey, medical record manager, is fairly new. She came straight from a college medical record program into the position; she is a quiet person, but knowledgeable and capable in a low-key manner.

Norman Richards, maintenance supervisor, is a long-time employee, and an exceptional all-around mechanic, but he exhibits a gruff, crude approach in interpersonal matters that frequently causes friction with employees. Richards's employees are also responsible for hospital security.

John Preston, chief laboratory technologist, runs a small but efficient laboratory operation. He has been in the position for six years.

Carol George, housekeeping supervisor, has been with Wilton more than 20 years and has been supervisor for more than 10 years. Her department's work is always top-notch, but you are frequently made aware of problems arising between housekeeping and nursing.

Patricia Conway, chief x-ray technologist, is a working supervisor, one of three people in the department. You have little contact with her, and problems with x-ray are rare.

Nancy Taylor, food service manager, has been at Wilton for eight years. Her department has the hospital's highest percentage of employee turnover and experiences the greatest number of disciplinary actions.

Cecil Leroy, pharmacist, is both "manager" and staff of a one-person department. You regard his work as of consistent high quality, and you feel the only problems that involve pharmacy are Leroy's occasional conflicts with nursing (usually over pharmacy hours).

Michael Shawn, purchasing agent, has been at Wilton for four years. He does all of the buying for the hospital except for certain food items. He is occasionally at odds with Mrs. Taylor over the extent of his involvement in buying for her department.

Today is Friday. Your secretary went home feeling ill less than one hour after reporting to work. You did not see her, however, because you had a meeting at 8:00 A.M. outside of the hospital and did not reach your office until 9:25 A.M.

When you entered your office you found a meeting notice and a short, handwritten note from administrator John Patrick. He had been called away suddenly, and he directed you to take his place at today's meeting of the Regional Hospital Association. You realize that you must leave no later than 10:00 A.M. to make the meeting, and, because the meeting will go on all afternoon and is some distance away, you will not be back in the office again until Monday.

Apparently, Sharon was at work long enough to assure that a number of items would await in your in-basket. You feel you need to get your in-basket under control before you leave.

Spend no more than 15 minutes reviewing the foregoing information and examining the organization chart (Figure 7–1). Then allow yourself 35 minutes to go through the in-basket and decide what must be done with each item. For each item, consider whether:

a. Action can—or must—be taken now, and what this action should be.
b. Action should be taken by others.
c. The item can, should, or must be postponed, and when it should be dealt with.
d. Some other course of action is called for.

Write out your intended response to each item in your in-basket. Your decisions regarding the items you decide to resolve at once should be expressed in the form of draft correspondence (notes or memorandums).

Figure 7–1 Partial Organization Chart

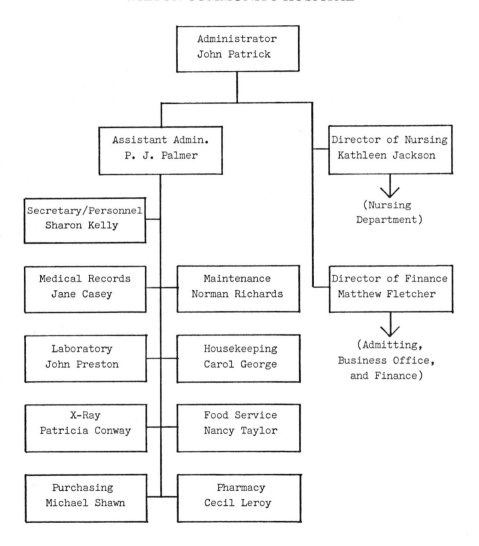

WILTON COMMUNITY HOSPITAL

MEMO

TO: All Departments

FROM: Administration

SUBJECT: Telephone Number Change

As you are aware, because of a misprint in last year's telephone directory the number for the administration office had to be changed from 234-2441 to 234-2440. The correct number—234-2440—was placed in this year's directory. However, because many outside callers apparently continue to use old directories there has been an increasing problem with a large number of general calls from the outside reaching the administration office directly instead of the switchboard.

To try to resolve this problem, the main number for administration is being changed back to 234-2441, and 234-2440 is being eliminated.

Please remove 2440 from your listings as administration's number and use 2441 from now on.

(Note)

P. J.—

Mrs. Taylor was looking for you first thing this morning. She claims that some of her kitchen workers have been approached by a pair of union organizers who have been promising them the moon. She also says she heard that the organizers have been talking to the housekeepers and maintenance men as well.

She thought you ought to know about it.

Sharon

(Telephone Message Slip)

To _P. J._

Date _Friday_   Time _8:20 a.m._

WHILE YOU WERE OUT

M _iss Jackson_

of _____

Phone _____

Area Code		Number	Extension

TELEPHONED	X	PLEASE CALL	X
CALLED TO SEE YOU		WILL CALL AGAIN	
WANTS TO SEE YOU		URGENT	
	RETURNED YOUR CALL	

Message _Didn't say what she wanted but asked if Mrs. George had been to see you yet about "an old common problem."_

_S._

Operator

(Note)

P. J. —

Both of the 3:00-to-11:00 maintenance men will be off today. Williams called in sick, and Powalski is still on vacation.

The large dishwasher is leaking badly, and Taylor is giving me fits. I can handle the dishwasher myself, but we are going to be stuck for security coverage on the second shift.

I might be able to cover by getting Carson to stay until 7:00 and bringing the night man in four hours early. Will you approve the overtime?

Norm

(Interruption)

Your telephone rings. On the third ring you remember that Sharon is not at her usual place, so you answer it yourself. It is the hospital's receptionist in the main lobby. She says to you:

"Sorry to interrupt you. I know Sharon's not there; otherwise, I'd be calling her directly.

"There's a salesman from some medical supply house out here at the desk. A Mr. Burton. Said he was passing through the area and remembered there was something he wanted to talk with you about. He asked for Mr. Shawn first, but Mike's in a meeting."

MEMO

TO: P. J. Palmer

FROM: Carol George

The nurses in the west wing have been telling my housekeepers what to do again. Every time I give an order I find that some nurse has handed out a different assignment. I am falling behind on routine cleaning, and my people don't know which way to turn.

It is about time we decided if housekeeping is run by me or by Miss Jackson's nurses.

(Telephone Message Slip)

To _P. J._

Date _Friday_   Time _9:05 a.m._

WHILE YOU WERE OUT

Mr. _John Preston_

of _____

Phone _____

| Area Code | Number | Extension |

TELEPHONED	X	PLEASE CALL	
CALLED TO SEE YOU		WILL CALL AGAIN	
WANTS TO SEE YOU		URGENT	
	RETURNED YOUR CALL		

Message _No message, but he says he needs to talk with you as soon as possible._

_S._

Operator

MEMO

TO: All Department Heads

FROM: Matt Fletcher, Director of Finance

SUBJECT: Equipment Inventory

A hospital-wide inventory of furniture and equipment must be completed by the end of the month (just ten days away). For every item assigned to your department we need:

- item description, such as standard desk, steno desk, electric typewriter, etc.;
- asset number—the four-digit number on a brass tag somewhere on the item;
- general condition.

You are likely to experience problems because of missing asset numbers and other difficulties, so you should consider this a high-priority requirement and get moving on it at once.

cc: P. J. Palmer
John Patrick

MEMO

TO: All Supervisors

FROM: Mike Shawn, Purchasing

SUBJECT: Min./Max. Stock

We are attempting to establish minimum and maximum stock levels for all nonmedical supplies that pass through the main storeroom. To do this, we need the following information from each of your departments:

- a list of the supplies you regularly draw through the storeroom;
- the usage rate of each item, in units per month;
- required minimum amount of each item to be available in the department.

I need this information no later than next Thursday noon. Thanks for your help.

cc: P. J. Palmer

MEMO

TO: P. J. Palmer
FROM: John Patrick, Administrator
SUBJECT: Possible Legal Action

I have been told that we are going to be sued by a patient who was supposedly injured when he fell against a housekeeping cart left in the doorway of his room.

I am unable to find an incident report, and nursing seems to know nothing about it. The mishap supposedly occurred on or about November 24.

Please fill me in on this at our administrative staff meeting this coming Tuesday.

cc: Kathleen Jackson

MEMO

TO: All Supervisors
FROM: Matt Fletcher, Director of Finance
SUBJECT: Time Card Problems

Our payroll section has recently learned of several instances of employees punching in and out for fellow employees.

Please remind all of your hourly employees that punching another employee's card is against the work rules clearly spelled out in the employee handbook. Also advise them that future infractions will be dealt with severely.

cc: John Patrick

(Letter)

P. J. Palmer
Assistant Administrator
Wilton Community Hospital
Wilton, New York

Dear P. J.:

I listened with interest to your presentation on "Reduced Absenteeism Through Employee Motivation" at the State Hospital Association's Annual Personnel and Labor Relations Conference last month. It occurred to me that you would be the ideal speaker for the kickoff meeting of the newly organized Personnel Directors Group of the Regional Hospital Association.

The meeting will be held on the evening of March 20, just about a month from now. Your topic could be anything related to personnel administration—except your absenteeism speech, since most of the region's personnel directors heard you at the state conference.

Please let me know your decision within a week, if possible. Should you choose to participate, I could use a tentative presentation title at the time you give me your answer.

I hope you will seriously consider this invitation to help us launch the new organization on a high note.

Sincerely,

Art

Arthur Wilson, Program Chairman
Regional Personnel Directors Group

(Interruption)

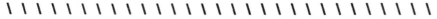

Your telephone rings again. This time you take it on the first ring. A high-pitched female voice says rapidly:

"You're Palmer? You're the boss today? The telephone lady said Patrick—that's who I wanted, John Patrick—isn't here so you're the boss today.

"I'm Mrs. Lulu Evanston, and I'm stuck here in room 135 because Ed Willoughby—that's Dr. Willoughby—doesn't know what he's doing. Never *did* know what he was doing, even in high school, as I recall.

"Anyway, I'm stuck here with nothing to do and some snippy little nurse won't tell me where my cigarettes are. Says Ed—Dr. Willoughby— won't let me smoke. But he never told *me* that, but that nurse won't listen. But you people will listen to my nephew Brian, I bet. He's on the hospital *board* and that sort of makes him *your* boss.

"And furthermore . . . ."

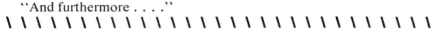

Chapter 8

Introduction to Questions

The questions presented in Chapter 9 are arranged in six groups reflecting the six combinations of primary focus and secondary focus used for classifying the cases. By far the greatest number of questions have *people* as their primary focus and *task* as their secondary focus.

No effort was made to classify the questions further by topic. Brief review of the questions will reveal that most are concerned with *communication* in conjunction with one or more additional topics. The additional topics, among them *change management, criticism and discipline, delegation, motivation, people problems, rules and policies,* reveal a clear pattern of interest on the part of supervisors who asked the questions. Most were concerned primarily with matters of interpersonal relations.

Some 83 percent of the questions in Chapter 9 emphasize interpersonal relations. The majority of these—59 percent of all questions—are concerned with relations with employees. Most of the remainder—22 percent of all questions—reflect supervisors' concerns for relations with higher management, mostly immediate supervisors.

USING THE QUESTIONS

Most of the questions presented in Chapter 9 are not answerable in any specific sense. However, every question is capable of stimulating productive exploration when considered in all of its implications.

The implications of any particular question may go well beyond the various facets of the problem presented. It is also necessary to examine the questioner's viewpoint and apparent assumptions and decide where that person is "coming from" in asking the question. The supervisor who claims an employee is doing something "wrong" may be proceeding on the implicit assumption that his or her own attitude or behavior is "right." This gives rise to a word of caution to apply in considering a question: In addition to considering the problem as it is presented, also consider the attitudes, assumptions, actions, and opinions of the supervisor who asked the question. Interpersonal problems are precisely that—*inter*personal. The supervisor cannot simply be seen as *dealing with* a problem; in most instances the supervisor must be seen as *part of* the problem.

AN EXAMPLE

Consider question number 5–03: "As a newly appointed supervisor, how can I succeed in pulling away from the people I have worked with for so long?" This question was presented for discussion to 20 supervisors at an informal supervisory skills development workshop. The group's comments are summarized in the following paragraphs.

Pulling Away

The work group is also a social group or, more accurately, a collection of several overlapping social groups of varying size and closeness of membership. Assuming you were a normally integrated group member, you had a number of relationships that coincided with or perhaps extended beyond the working relationships you required in doing your work. Your peers were not simply your coworkers; some were your friends and most were your acquaintances. Undoubtedly you were closer to some than to others, and some you did not like as well as you liked certain others.

When you were selected from the group and appointed supervisor the structure of the group was altered and your membership in the group changed. Therefore, some "pulling away" began almost at once without your conscious effort to establish distance between you and the others. Structural changes and the change in your status were sufficient to cause some members of the group to begin pulling away from you. You are now "the boss," and whether or not the others willingly accept that fact, most of them will nevertheless recognize that you now have some authority which you did not previously possess and that your use of this authority could affect them and their jobs.

Your former peers, now your employees, may begin to pull away from you for a number of reasons:

- As mentioned, you are now an authority figure.
- To a few employees who will always regard "management" with suspicion, you are now "the enemy."
- Some employees may feel that because they got along well with you they will be the first ones you think of when there is extra work to be done.
- Some employees who considered you their friend may deliberately back away to avoid creating the appearance that they are trying to trade on your friendship.

To a number of employees, however, it is likely to be business as usual and socializing as usual regardless of your new role of supervisor. With some of the employees you may have to take deliberate steps intended to limit the extent of your relationships. It is easy for the appearance of favoritism to develop out of your relationship with a few employees. While you may be able to maintain such relationships and at the same time avoid playing favorites, it is often the *appearance* of favoritism that does the damage.

Some of your pulling away will also be encouraged by the effects of structural changes on you and the way you work. You now spend less time on the job with your former peers and considerably less time doing the actual hands-on work of the department. Rather, you are now required to spend a certain amount of time with other supervisors and higher managers, and it is also necessary to get involved in such management tasks as planning, scheduling, budgeting, performance appraisal, etc., which either keep you from contact with individual employees or channel some of your contacts along fairly specific lines. You must go your way while your employees continue to go theirs. Although your way and their way coincide much of the time (you have common departmental objectives) you nevertheless now have things to do which take you away from the group's immediate interests much of the time.

Management is often described as a lonely calling. This is true to some extent even at the level of the first-line supervisor. You no longer have your former full-fledged membership in the social groups that overlay the work group. Certain formerly close relationships are bound to be affected, and you cannot help feeling that you have lost something. Although by becoming a supervisor you supposedly opened the door to other relationships and membership in other groups, you have not gained to an extent that covers your losses. The departmental work group, because of its members' need to spend much time together in pursuit of common goals, encourages close and sometimes long-term relationships. However, the supervisory "group" is another matter. Supervisors, scattered throughout the organization, are each concerned with their own departments, and relationships among supervisors are often necessarily looser and less active than relationships among nonmanagers. Thus the lonely or isolated feeling—you no longer can be as close as you once were to your former friends and acquaintances, and your opportunities to form new close ties are limited.

As a supervisor promoted from the group you probably have a few more advantages than a supervisor recruited from outside of the institution. You know the organization and how its parts work together, you know the department and its tasks, and you know the people in the department. Probably the principal disadvantage you face is the tendency of many of your employees to remember you as "one of the gang." How well your entry into supervision is accepted by the other employees will depend to a considerable extent on how well you were regarded in the group before your promotion. If you were reasonably well liked and respected as a group member, then the employees will likely give you a reasonable chance to win their respect as supervisor.

Being liked is important to most of us; certainly we would rather be liked than disliked. However, in their desire to get along with everyone many supervisors make this mistake of putting the desire to be liked *first*. It is far better for the supervisor to be *respected*—respected for knowledge, integrity, fairness—than simply to be liked. You will be well on the way toward earning your employees' respect if you can convince them through your actions that you consider each an individual worthy of respect and special attention, but that your first priority—in fact, the first priority of the entire department—lies in fulfilling the department's objectives of service to the institution's patients.

To pull away from the group properly when you are appointed supervisor:

- Play fair. Go out of your way to assure that each employee receives equal consideration in all matters.
- Recognize that there is nothing you can do to guarantee that you will be liked by all employees at all times.
- Through your actions, strive to earn the respect of each employee. Don't assume that the limited respect which may be given your *position* is automatically owing to you as a person.
- Do not get carried away by the symbols of status and position.
- Recognize that your status as a group member has changed.
- Make sure you are simply pulling away, stepping back rather than turning around. You must remain visible and available to your employees. Your employees do not work *for* you so much as they work *with* you, and your primary function is to help them do their jobs as efficiently and effectively as possible.

Chapter 9

Questions from Health Care Supervisors

GROUP 1

Primary Focus: PEOPLE
Secondary Focus: TASK

A. Relations with Employees

1A–01: How can I tell an employee who is "never wrong" that he *is* in fact wrong?

1A–02: How should I handle an employee who becomes disturbed and resentful when reprimanded?

1A–03: How should a supervisor handle the criticism or disciplining of a usually good employee?

1A–04: What should I do with an employee who continues to repeat mistakes after having been spoken to about them several times?

1A–05: Are there any criteria for determining how long a person who has been criticized or unfavorably reviewed should be given for correction or improvement?

1A–06: I have an employee, a member of a minority group, who responds to all criticism, all attempts to delegate tasks, and most normal work instructions with charges of prejudice. How can I deal with this?

1A–07: How can I handle a particular employee who cannot take criticism like an adult? Every time I correct her she becomes defensive and immediately asks if this is going to go on her next evaluation.

1A–08: I have an employee who gives me cause for criticism by committing frequent errors in work procedure. No matter how soft I make the criticism—and I know this person's thin-skinned nature, so I try to be as tactful as possible—the reaction is always an abrupt denial of any wrongdoing. I could cite many specific incidents, but I have not done so because they do not leave much room for tact. However, I seem to be getting nowhere because I am failing to pin down the employee. Should I use the specific information available to me?

1A–09: How can I get the employees of one ward to conform to the rules of the building? This group never gets reports done on time, the ward appears disorganized and messy, and employees eat in the offices and treatment rooms. There are three wards in the building, but all of the problems are concentrated in this one group.

1A–10: What can the supervisor do to motivate the borderline employee?

1A–11: What can I do with an employee who I know can do better but refuses to try?

1A–12: A particular employee has one thing in his job he simply dislikes doing. How can I talk him into liking it?

1A–13: What kind of incentives can I use to get an employee to accomplish work more neatly while still turning out the quality required of the job?

1A–14: What can I do to better motivate the people on my staff, to get them to care about what they are doing and about their future within their profession?

1A–15: What is the best way to evaluate the motivators for a given group of employees, to determine what factors are most important in getting these particular people to perform?

1A–16: How can I encourage an employee to participate more fully in the activities of the department when she is apparently satisfied with what she has been doing?

1A–17: How can I permanently eliminate the attitude that causes people to respond to a request or a problem with: "That's not my responsibility (or my job, my floor, my department, etc.)"?

1A–18: How can I motivate my employees to adopt my way of thinking? I have worked their jobs myself, and I have found my ways to be best, but I cannot convince them of this.

1A–19: A certain employee of mine has a steady pace—slow. He accomplishes only about half the work of other people doing the same job, but when I talk with him he seems convinced he is doing his very best. I know he is capable of doing more, but how can I get him to do it?

1A–20: How can I get a crew of very unmotivated people motivated? I try to get them to take an interest in what they are doing and to carry out their jobs with concern for quality, but I find that I have to go out of my way to make them think they are doing it themselves rather than being coerced into it.

1A–21: I have a fairly high percentage of younger nurses on my floor. I often get the feeling that many of them are just putting in their time— three to five years or so—before deciding to start families or move on to something else. Most of my attempts at delegating short-term projects generate no enthusiasm or willing involvement, although I have made several serious attempts. How can I motivate these people, or better still, get them to be self-motivated?

1A–22: How can I get an employee to do a particular task when all the signals I am getting suggest that the employee thinks I should really be doing this task myself?

1A–23: How can I deal with an employee who refuses to do delegated work? This person seems to have complete disregard for authority.

1A–24: What is a good response to the employee who asks, "Why should I?", or says, "It's not part of my job," when asked to do something. I find that the answer, "Because I said so," usually produces no results and often generates hostility.

1A–25: How should I handle an employee who seems unwilling to do what he is told? Whenever I give him an order he decides that something else is more important. He usually does what he has decided, leaving me to discover later that what I had requested has not even been started.

1A–26: How can I handle a hot-tempered employee without blowing up myself?

1A–27: How can I deal with a hotheaded employee who seems to take everything I say the wrong way?

1A–28: How should I handle an employee who seems to have decided she is not going to do as asked without creating a scene?

1A–29: What should I do with an employee who behaves flippantly over an error which is potentially quite serious?

1A–30: I have several employees who seem unable or unwilling to do things as I expect them to be done. How can I get these people to follow instructions?

1A–31: How can I work with a know-it-all employee who always seems to take a stand in direct opposition to mine?

1A–32: How do I deal with an employee who works well alone but who communicates poorly and causes problems with other employees?

1A–33: What can I do about an employee who is effective when on the job but who cannot be depended upon to show up when scheduled to work on weekends?

1A–34: How can I direct commands to an employee who was in charge of my department before I came on the scene without causing hard feelings?

1A–35: How can I deal with a willing employee who is extremely inconsistent in her work? Sometimes she is quite good, but just as often she is careless and forgetful.

1A–36: How do I communicate with an employee who is closed to suggestions, fights the facts, and even in normal conversation always claims to "know it all"?

1A–37: How can I get through to an employee who has such a one-track mind that even written proof is denied? Her attitude seems to be: "Don't confuse me with facts—my mind is made up."

1A–38: How can I get a particular employee to see my point of view? She seems blind to all views except her own, but I know without a doubt that she is wrong.

1A–39: What is the best way to go about establishing a relationship with an employee who now has me as a supervisor after working for more than ten years without direct supervision?

1A–40: How should I approach a reasonably intelligent and effective employee who appears neat and well groomed, but whose personal hygiene is offensive to other employees?

1A–41: What can I do to increase the productivity of an older employee who has been removed from a position of authority and must now work alongside employees she formerly supervised?

1A–42: One of my employees, an average performer, is assigned one task she so dislikes that she complains about it every time it comes up and avoids it whenever she possibly can. How can I talk her into liking it?

1A–43: What can I do with an employee who is constantly interfering in other people's business and always making waves, and whose behavior often borders on insubordination? This same employee is skilled and knowledgeable and delivers excellent patient care.

1A–44: What can I do with an employee whose tactlessness and general negative attitude have a terrible effect on relationships with coworkers? Her peers seem to dislike her to the point of trying to avoid working with her most of the time.

1A–45: How can I deal with several employees who seem unable to differentiate between criticism on a professional level and on a personal level? Almost without fail every bit of job-related criticism I offer is taken as a personal attack.

1A–46: I have an employee who seems to feel that she is the only one in the department who is fully capable of doing any job that comes up. She continually finds fault with whatever anyone else does and is always making trouble for her coworkers. How can I handle this employee?

1A–47: I have an employee who complains constantly about getting the more complicated patients and claims that another employee gets only easier patients because she cannot handle sick people. She is quick to point out that she and the other employee both receive the same pay but are not doing equal work. What can I say to the complaining employee?

1A–48: Should I try to convince an employee who is older than the voluntary retirement age but still younger than the mandatory retirement age that he should retire? He seems convinced that he is pulling his weight, but that is far from correct. My head says he should go, but my heart is not so sure.

1A–49: I have a new employee who seems unable to take the probationary process seriously. He jokes about his mistakes and makes no apparent effort to correct them, and he bends while not quite breaking all of the work rules. He seems unaware that everything he is doing is leading toward termination at the end of the probation period. How can I wake him up?

1A–50: I cannot seem to get through to a certain employee. She talks very little, even to the point of avoiding direct questions, and when I give her an instruction she simply stares at me for a moment before going about her business. I know she is capable of doing better work, but her performance has not improved one particle in the three years she has been on the staff. What can I do about this employee?

1A–51: How can a supervisor deal with an employee who may have genuine personality problems? The erratic behavior of one particular employee is affecting my whole department; this employee experiences abrupt mood changes and bounces between sweetness and light and doom and gloom in the same hour. Also, this employee is extremely sensitive to criticism and becomes argumentative over the smallest matter.

1A–52: I have an employee who frequently expresses the belief that he is overqualified for the position he holds. Considering his advanced education and experience, he may indeed be overqualified. However, he makes no effort to look into any of the positions opening up here at the medical center, and as far as I know he has not investigated opportunities elsewhere. He seems to be feeding his own discontent by prolonging his stay on a job in which he is underutilized and bored. Is there anything I can do for him—or *with* him?

1A–53: We have a problem with overstaffing on the day shift in some of the nursing units. Yet we are short-staffed on evenings and nights. We do not seem able to find many people willing to work anything but days. One of my employees—a good worker, but having the least seniority in the group—was just told she must be reassigned to nights. She says she cannot work nights because of transportation problems, and she will have to quit if we insist. Nursing administration will not retract the order because the transfer would then fall to the next lowest in seniority, and this person could file a grievance and win. Is there any way to manage this situation so a good employee will not be lost?

1A–54: How can a supervisor control gossip?

1A–55: How should I handle friction between employees?

1A–56: How can I deal with two employees who do not get along without seeming to favor one or the other?

1A–57: What can I do with two employees who are constantly aggravating each other? On numerous occasions each has complained to me about the other.

1A–58: I am often asked to help with personal problems that develop between employees and sometimes between fellow supervisors. Is it my place to try to deal with such problems?

1A–59: Two employees in my department are engaged in a long-running battle. I have hesitated to get too deeply involved for fear of making both parties angry with me. What should I do?

1A–60: The personality differences among three people in my department affect the work of the entire department. Besides talking directly with the persons involved, what can I do?

1A–61: I know there are going to be personality conflicts; not everyone gets along equally well with everyone else, and some people simply rub each other the wrong way. But what can I do about a personality conflict that is having a negative effect on my entire department?

1A–62: How can I handle a few employees who constantly backbite and gossip about each other? These people all work on the same floor, and none can easily be transferred. I have talked with them as a group and have spoken sternly with the worst offenders on a one-to-one basis. Nothing has helped. Presently I ignore all the griping from this group, yet I realize that this is certainly no solution.

1A–63: A fairly straightforward task usually performed by one employee was delegated to another for a two-day period during which the regularly assigned person was absent. The fill-in employee did the best she could do under the circumstances, but the person who usually did the work was highly critical of the way it was done while she was away. Who should I be criticizing—the one who may have mishandled the task, the one who took it upon herself to criticize a fellow employee, or both?

1A–64: I have two employees who were both clearly interested in promotion to a newly created job involving a small amount of supervisory responsibility. The two were never particularly friendly, and now the one who did not get the job shows signs of jealousy toward the promoted person. The one who missed out on the promotion has made it plain to the rest of the staff that she feels the promotion should have been hers, and I am afraid that the tone of uneasiness spreading among the staff will have a serious effect on morale. How can I deal with this?

1A–65: Our medication procedures require the night staff to check all medicine tickets against the original physicians' orders every night to assure that proper medication is being provided. Recently a physician's order was transferred incorrectly on the day shift, and the incorrect medication was administered for three consecutive days. A brief check revealed that over the course of the three days, five night shift people had signed off the check-sheet indicating that all medicine tickets had been checked and found to be correct. What should be done about this?

1A–66: Two employees in my department both feel they should be given more responsibility when I am absent. Both are extremely competent workers. One, however, has been my backup for several years and does a commendable job. The other employee is "knocking on the door," so to speak, displaying willingness to accept more responsibility. I am perfectly satisfied with my backup person, but I do not want to see the other employee's obvious enthusiasm dampened. How can I handle this without hurting either employee?

1A–67: When I returned to the hospital after a two-day conference an employee sought me out and told me that an important task to which she and a coworker were assigned did not get done because the coworker took advantage of my absence to coast for a couple of days. The other party, when asked about the assignment, rattled off a lengthy list of excuses— minor emergencies, unexpected requests, and other interruptions, none of which could readily be verified. I am left with two completely different stories and an important job still undone. Where do I go from here?

1A–68: Is there any advice to help me in doing performance appraisals on several people I have worked with for a long time? These employees are my contemporaries in years. We have spent a long time as friends and coworkers, but thanks to a recent promotion I am now the supervisor.

1A–69: How can I accomplish complete performance appraisal when there is no money available for pay raises?

1A–70: Should employees be required to sign their performance evaluations?

1A–71: As a supervisor I have certain administrative functions that take me away from the department and its immediate problems. My absence seems to produce negative reactions in my employees, as if they are telling me I am not doing my job because I am not around when they need me. How can I deal with this?

1A–72: How should I handle an assistant who continuously seems to be trying to usurp my authority?

B. Relations with Higher Management

1B–01: How can I relate to a manager who does not listen to the supervisors who work for him? All input and feedback from the lower management—questions and problems, solutions, ideas for running the department—seem to fall on deaf ears.

1B–02: I have a problem that I cannot deal with because it is clearly beyond the limits of my authority. I have approached my boss about it with all the details and even with suggestions for how it might be resolved, but no correction has been attempted. What can I do next?

1B–03: Every time I take a problem to my boss it gets thrown back at me; I am told to deal with it myself or take it to someone else, or else I am asked to suggest what I would do and that becomes the answer. What am I really up against, and how can I deal with it?

1B–04: How does a supervisor get higher management to follow through on problems that desperately need attention?

1B–05: I have an employee problem that needs immediate attention for the sake of the entire department, but I cannot awaken higher management to the urgency of the situation. What should I do?

1B–06: My boss recently told me to have my employees do something to which I am opposed. I disagreed, and I am sure she could see I was quite upset about it, but she was in a hurry and refused to listen. What recourse do I have?

1B–07: As head nurse it is my job to do what my supervisor tells me to do. But how can I successfully push a new program my supervisor has directed me to implement when the charge nurse who works for me is opposed to it?

1B–08: How can a supervisor deal with a department head who does not provide backup on disciplinary actions concerning employees?

1B–09: I have a night-shift employee whose performance is unsatisfactory. She has been caught sleeping on the job several times. I reprimanded her each time, and the nursing office has issued a written warning. However, our system forbids dismissal without the approval of administration and employee relations, and neither has responded. This has been going on for months, and the employee is making no effort to improve. How can I get action?

1B-10: At my request, my immediate manager gave me permission to deal with another department's supervisor on an important and sensitive matter. He explained that he could not be available, but that I could act with every assurance of his backing regardless of the outcome.

I proceeded. The matter turned out to be more sensitive that even I had imagined, and there were serious repercussions. Now I have to face the consequences alone; it seems my manager has conveniently forgotten our conversation, and the backing I was counting on will not be forthcoming. Where can I go from here?

1B-11: It has been said that creativity is one of the supervisor's best defenses against stagnation. But what can the supervisor with creative tendencies do when the immediate boss seems to stifle or even punish creativity?

1B-12: I have made it a point to learn a great deal about the team approach to nursing, and I would like to try it in my unit. However, nursing administration, which is actually quite distant from the delivery of patient care at this institution, is completely unfamiliar with the concept. How can I go about selling the team approach to nursing administration?

1B-13: My boss often deals directly with my employees without going through me. How can I get the boss to communicate in such a way that I do not lose the respect of my subordinates?

1B-14: I have supervisory responsibility for eight employees, and I think I know how to do my job, yet my boss is practically in my pocket for eight hours a day reminding, pointing, nudging, correcting, and suggesting. What can I do about this overbossing?

1B-15: How can I deal with a boss who has made it plain that she expects to be informed in detail of a situation I consider to be highly confidential?

1B-16: How can an assistant supervisor handle complaints against the supervisor without either joining in the complaining or seeming not to care? Should one manager make excuses for another manager with the employees?

1B-17: How can I keep myself from being trapped in the middle when dealing with two different bosses?

1B-18: How can I handle a situation in which there is a broad division of authority because of one higher manager's chronic absence and apparent lack of interest?

1B-19: We are in a period of reorganization of the administrative staff, and four of the five top administrative positions will change hands within the next 90 days. Members of the middle management group seem to communicate effectively and get along well. How can we maintain middle management's working relationships in the face of massive administrative change?

1B–20: A particular management position was eliminated in a shake-up of the medical center's management structure. The affected manager, apparently well liked by administration, had only a short time left before retirement so he was given another management position at the same level. The new position, however, required knowledge and skills completely different from those required in the manager's former position. The people in the present manager's department used to work together as an effective team. However, this manager is closed to employee input and suggestions, will not accept many methods that have already been proven, and is generally inflexible. What lies in store for this department?

1B–21: As a middle manager, how can I—or how dare I—tell administration that their actions are the greatest cause of fear and unrest in the organization? I do not believe they see the apprehension they instill by their failure to communicate and by their tendency to surround most of their planning and decision making with secrecy.

1B–22: What can a supervisor do to improve staff morale when all such efforts are constantly undermined by the actions of administration?

C. Relations with Others

1C–01: We have a training program which all nonprofessional nursing staff who administer medication must complete. Several employees took the program two to three years ago, but now inservice education claims they are unable to find any records of this particular class. Inservice has requested the employees to repeat the course for proper certification. Most of them do not want to do it, and a few have said they consider the request unfair and unreasonable. Most of the employees involved are good workers, and their morale has been good—until now, anyway. What can we do to keep from losing some of these people?

1C–02: There seems to be plenty of effective communication between administration and nursing, but many other departments, especially the smaller ones, are left out when it comes to learning of changes in policies and procedures and even changes in management personnel. How can the voices of the smaller departments be heard over nursing?

1C–03: Most of our organizational units behave more like competitors and independent empires than departments of the institution. How can we make individual departments realize that each is a necessary part of the whole, but that none alone is the most important?

GROUP 2

Primary Focus: PEOPLE
Secondary Focus: SELF

A. Relations with Employees

2A–01: What is the best way to handle my employees' criticism of the way I run my department?

2A–02: What can a supervisor do about genuine personality clashes between supervisor and employee?

2A–03: Is there an acceptable approach to delegating authority without making subordinates feel that the work is simply being pushed off on them?

2A–04: Is it possible to be an effective supervisor and still be everybody's friend?

2A–05: I think it is only natural that I like certain people in the group more than others, but this presents me with hazards as a supervisor. How can I guard against becoming partial to some employees?

2A–06: A certain supervisor, recently promoted to the position, seems reluctant to criticize or even comment on the work of his subordinates. He appears to want to remain the "nice guy." How can he be an effective supervisor and appropriately evaluate his employees? Will he be likely to change through time and experience?

B. Relations with Higher Management

2B–01: How do I get to see a higher manager who is always too busy for me? Notes and telephone calls are no use; the notes never get answered and the phone calls do not get through.

2B–02: My department head is always too busy to listen when I have questions, problems, or suggestions. When I try to get a moment of her time she invariably says, "Get back to you in a minute," and then takes off and that is the end of it. How can I relate to a boss like this?

2B–03: As a supervisor, what can I do to make my department head more receptive to suggestions?

2B–04: How can I deal with an authoritarian department head—a virtual dictator—who has less skill, less training, and less seniority than I have?

2B–05: I have to work for two bosses who are diametrically opposed on almost everything. It is especially difficult for me to get backing on disciplinary actions—one boss is a harsh disciplinarian, and the other is soft. How can I possibly deal effectively with my employees under such conditions?

2B–06: As a supervisor I rarely get cooperation or backing from my manager. It has been this way since I was first promoted to supervisor. In fact, administration promoted me without my manager even knowing about it. The manager acts as though I do not exist. How can I perform my duties under these conditions?

2B–07: Is it appropriate for a manager to request that his reporting relationship be switched from one administrative representative to another?

GROUP 3

Primary Focus: TASK
Secondary Focus: PEOPLE

3–01: How good is a manager who selects people he believes can do the job with minimal assistance and then watches over them carefully until the work is done to his satisfaction?

3–02: How long should staff meetings last, and in what setting should they be held?

3–03: As supervisor of the business office I work Monday through Friday. However, two of the positions reporting to me have to be staffed seven days a week. My employees rotate to cover Saturdays and Sundays; they are qualified to do the work, and they know they can call me if problems arise. However, I have heard some grumbling about my failure to work weekends. Should I assume a share of weekend duty for the sake of harmony in the department?

3–04: We do evaluations of employees every three months, and I want to know why. Work performance, if it is good, does not seem to change much; it is usually the same, evaluation after evaluation. Is the evaluation process a waste of time?

3–05: Why does our institution tend to use length of service as the main qualification for promotion, rather than using employee capability as the main criterion?

3–06: Should it be the supervisor or the hospital's personnel director who has the final word in departmental hiring?

3–07: Recently my department was forced into sharing the same physical space with another department. We have encountered some terrible adjustment problems. How can we help the employees of both departments adjust successfully instead of simply "making the best of a bad situation" (as administration told us to do)?

3–08: I do not have enough weekend help to keep my unit running the way it should. My people are overworked, and their morale is crumbling, but the only answer I get from the front office is, "There is nobody we can send you." What can I do?

GROUP 4

Primary Focus: TASK
Secondary Focus: SELF

4–01: In the maintenance department it seems that most of the problems are emergencies. It is extremely difficult to delegate properly and allocate one's time because the emergencies change whatever momentum had existed. How can a supervisor possibly manage time under these conditions?

4–02: What can I do to make evening, night, and weekend staffing easier?

4–03: As a registered nurse and working supervisor, I was transferred from an interesting job to a dead-ended, intellectually numbing position in a department where people are encouraged to spy on each other and report the commission of such sins as using black ink instead of blue ink on medication records. This may sound small, but it happened. We were temporarily out of blue pens, so I fell back on the only thing I could find — black. In such a situation should I (1) refuse to chart, (2) swipe someone else's blue pen; (3) cry? Seriously, what should I do?

GROUP 5

Primary Focus: TASK
Secondary Focus: PEOPLE

5–01: Is it possible for me to change the opinions of my coworkers once they have come to believe that I am too easygoing?

5–02: When being liked by subordinates is important, what is the best approach for the supervisor to follow in administering disciplinary action?

5–03: As a newly appointed supervisor, how can I succeed in pulling away from the people I have worked with for so long?

5–04: I am about to become supervisor of a group of people who have worked together for years. All these people know the department's several jobs well, and I know these jobs hardly at all. Also, I have never before worked in a supervisory capacity. Is there any advice that will help me get started on the right foot?

5–05: I am young and I am new to professional nursing and new to the hospital, but I have already been placed in charge of a nursing unit. I am comfortable with my nursing knowledge, but I am uneasy with management and I do not think I handle authority very well. Even the cleaning lady on the unit talks back and argues when I speak with her, apparently because she is older and has been there longer. How can I make any headway under such circumstances?

5–06: How can I handle a pushy salesman who has the knack of dropping in on my busiest days?

GROUP 6

Primary Focus: SELF
Secondary Focus: TASK

6–01: How can the supervisor who comes up through the ranks learn how to relate on different levels on the way up?

6–02: How does the leader who has been promoted from the ranks best adjust to the supervisory role?

6–03: Why should I avoid giving in to the temptation to do a particular job myself rather than delegate it when I know that in the long run this would be easier?

6–04: What can be done about supervisors who do not seem to see themselves as instructors as well as managers?

6–05: Should every supervisor or manager have a private office?

6–06: How can I turn my mind off and leave my problems at the hospital rather than take them home with me?

Chapter 10

What Can You Get from All This?

PRACTICE

The conscientious use of case studies provides you with practice in analyzing problems and making decisions. A case is not the "real world," of course, so true decision-making pressures and emotional involvement in the decision situation are missing. However, there is a plus side to even these apparent shortcomings of the case method—you can practice decision-making techniques without doing any damage through a few "wrong" decisions.

Since a real-world decision includes personal involvement, potential consequences, and often the pressure of time, a case study cannot simulate all of the moves required in making and implementing a decision. However, a case study allows you to go through some of the necessary moves and thus more closely parallels reality than does a simple recounting of rules or principles. In one important way, decision making is like many other human endeavors—the more you practice, the more proficient you become.

NEW PROBLEM-SOLVING OUTLOOK

Although a case is not reality, it nevertheless demonstrates the complexity of the real decision-making environment. Dealing with a case requires that you retreat from theory and other abstractions and face the uncertainties of the real world. Through the case study method you learn to make necessary simplifications, to cut through a maze of apparent facts and information and create a working order that you can deal with in a practical way.

No single case ever supplies "all of the facts." In dealing with a case, just as in pondering many real-life situations, it is always possible to ask, "What if . . .?" But rarely does the supervisor have "all of the facts" in any but the simplest of situations.

Trying to decide without full knowledge of a situation is often frustrating, but this is part of the supervisory task. If there were fewer such frustrations there would likely be fewer difficult decisions to make, and fewer supervisors required to make them.

In spite of the shortcomings of the case study method, however, conscientiously working your way through a number of case studies can leave you with a new outlook on problem solving. This new outlook may well include your recognition of the need to:

- thoroughly evaluate all the information you have available, and arrange bits of information in some priority order;
- arrange your information into meaningful patterns or decision alternatives;
- evaluate each alternative according to the objectives to be served by the decision;
- make a choice.

Rarely is there a single "right" solution to a given case. More often than not it is even difficult to say whether one particular answer is better than another. In this respect, however, the case study method supports reality—in real-world situations what is "right" is usually relative to the conditions of the moment and the needs of the people involved.

The use of the case study method also reminds us of the true role of rules, principles, and theories. We quickly discover that rules, principles, and theories are but the tools we work with and not the ends we are trying to serve. We learn to arrange information so we can use our tools as they are needed, rather than attempt to organize our case analyses around the tools. In other words, we learn that theory *serves* practice—it does not *dictate* practice.

To help you decide for yourself whether you are getting something from the use of the case study method, try to assess your "answer" to each case you complete according to the following questions:

- Do my recommendations show that I fully understand the issues involved in the case?

- Given the absence of unforeseen circumstances, could my recommendations realistically solve the problem? That is, are they workable under the circumstances?
- Do my recommendations appear to be as fair as possible to all parties involved in the problem?
- Do my recommendations support the goals of the organization rather than the goals of some specific person or group?
- If this were not a case but rather a real problem, could I live with my recommendations?

BROADENED VIEW

The advantages of the case study method are never more apparent than when cases are considered by a group of persons working together. The multiple inputs provided by group activity serve as a strong stimulus to creativity. Ideas lead to more ideas; another person may mention an idea that had not occurred to you, and this in turn can lead you to think of something that neither of you had mentioned. Ideas—implications, possibilities, what have you—build upon ideas, and often the thought that leads to a sound solution springs from discussion of peripheral issues or matters of yet-to-be-recognized importance. Much of the time, group consideration of a case reveals more potentially productive alternatives than one person would have generated alone.

Also, different persons viewing the same case will bring different viewpoints to bear. Each of us possesses a unique viewpoint, that being the sum of our own attitudes, experience, background, etc. We are inclined to view the same problem in different ways; we will see some factors as more important than others because of the way we are put together.

Consider, for instance, a problem concerning a request for more housekeeping personnel arising during a period of financial restraint. To the finance director the dollar problems may loom as the most significant issue in the overall problem. However, the housekeeping supervisor, struggling with an overworked and understaffed department, will perhaps see understaffing as the critical issue. And even without professional involvement in the problem, any two supervisors from different disciplines may well view things differently. The same hypothetical problem—the housekeeping staffing situation—may be viewed in two completely different ways by, say, a registered nurse and a laboratory technologist.

Differing views come from different orientations. You alone stand in a unique spot in the organization, so no one else views all things quite the same way you do. No department exists in isolation from all others in the delivery of health care, and there are few kinds of problems that do not cross departmental lines, so the views of a number of people of varying backgrounds usually contribute to the development of more numerous and comprehensive alternatives.

Group participation in case study activity also points up the need for compromise in problem solving. Again reminded that few activities and few problems in a health organization are isolated from each other, any decision rendered usually has to accommodate more than one particular interest. We find that our need becomes not that of developing the "best" solution, one which may be "best" logically and economically although it may serve the desires of one interested party, but rather developing a solution that is fair and workable overall, one that serves the objectives of the organization rather than the desires of an individual.

THE BENEFITS OF THE CASE METHOD

In summary, the case study method of learning provides the following benefits:

- practice in idea generation and creative problem solving;
- familiarization with logical problem-solving processes;
- broadened perspective, owing to the sharing of ideas and viewpoints with others;
- encouragement in developing the habit of approaching problems analytically;
- some limited "practice" in solving problems and making decisions.

As mentioned in Chapter 1, the case study method is but one of several methods available for presenting supervisory development material. No supervisor's continuing education should rely 100 percent on the case method; many things—specific rules, principles, and techniques, for instance—are best acquired by other means. However, the case method has characteristics that make it worth consideration as a significant part of a supervisor's continuing education: It calls for the active involvement of the supervisor in the learning process, and it significantly narrows the gap between theory and practice.

Chapter 11

Collecting Your Own Cases

SOURCES OF CASE MATERIAL

One excellent source of material for cases is your own experience. Many items suitable for case presentation can be found in experiences you have had in your present position and in jobs you held in the past.

Hardly a day goes by in which each working supervisor could not point to at least one or two instances which could be written up as cases. Such things happen to all of us day in and day out. However, most potential cases slide by us; only the truly troublesome matters remain clearly in mind after the fact. Of course, the big problems, those we remember clearly, make excellent cases, but so do many of the smaller matters which we deal with and forget.

If you want to collect case material, your conscious decision to do so will probably remind you to remain alert for opportunities. When something happens that may later make a useful case, make note of it, briefly but in sufficient detail to allow you to recall the incident when you need to.

Even a relatively new supervisor's brief experience—say, three or four months or so—can furnish many useful cases. None of these cases may be truly original as far as the issues they deal with are concerned, but each is likely to have unique implications.

Remaining with your experience for a moment, another excellent source of case material—quite likely the best available source—is your mistakes, those perhaps painful occasions when you "learned the hard way." If you made a mistake, recognized that you erred, and benefited from the experience, then it is likely that you have the issues clearly in mind. It is also likely that you know something about the cause of the error, why the mistake was indeed a mistake.

You may also find case material in your observations of the actions of other people, people you have worked for, those who have reported to you, and others whose working lives have touched yours. You can use secondhand information as well, stories of the experiences of other supervisors.

You can also fabricate cases completely from scratch. Start with a basic question, especially one on the order of, "What should I do *if* . . .?" and build a brief tale that describes the problem acted out rather than expressed as a question. Many of the questions contained in Chapter 9, "Questions from Health Care Supervisors," can be used in this fashion. In fact, four or five of the cases used in the *Casebook* were generated in this fashion. If a supervisor asks, for instance, "What can I do with an ordinarily good employee who will not take orders from one particular head nurse?" you can certainly make up a two- or three-paragraph "short story" featuring an employee's refusal to respond to a supervisor's orders.

FACT IN FICTIONAL FORM

When writing up cases based on actual events, be sure to fictionalize your material. Write in such a way that no actual person can be identified. Do not name specific institutions known to you—especially your own institution—and never describe an actual organization, department, or other setting so accurately that the people involved can be identified without being named. Make up names for your characters, and you should indeed consider them to be characters, just as though you were writing fiction.

Invent names for institutions, and consider altering institutional characteristics such as size, affiliation, and elements of organizational structure to obscure the source of your material further.

If an actual happening you would like to use as a case proves to be unique, to be so odd, unusual, or dramatic that the participants could still be identified no matter how they were disguised, then forget it. It is better to let even an excellent example go untapped than to run the risk of invading someone's privacy.

For each case you propose to write you should be able to pose the central issue, that is, the main problem, or the topic of the case, in the form of a single, relatively concise question. Most of the questions in Chapter 9 can be related by theme to various cases. For instance, Question 1A–22 ("How can I get an employee to do a particular task when all the signals I am getting suggest that the employee thinks I should really be doing this task myself?'') advances the central issue of Case P/S–05–02 (''It's His Job, Not Mine''). Having thus clearly identified the central issue, proceed to weave your fictional tale to show the development of the issue in a few words (as opposed to simply restating the issue).

KEEP IT SIMPLE

Simplify your material, sticking to just those things you need to develop the issue at the heart of the case appropriately. In none but the most elementary supervisory problems can we hope to capture all of the available information; in most instances we cannot do so without generating cases that are far too long and complicated for practical use. This is especially true of problems concerning people. There are many sides to most people problems and much of the available information is subjective.

Sticking to the central issue, provide a few pertinent facts. Also, if you believe it would be helpful—as it usually is in cases involving people problems—insert a few words of observation or insight relative to a participant's characteristics or manner of behavior. An example of this appears in Case P/T–13–05 (''The Voice'') in which a person is described as having a ''loud, screechy, irritating voice.'' A bit of this kind of character description can provide the user of the case with some insight into the kinds of human relations problems that might be involved.

In general, the depth of information used in a case should be such that the reader can clearly identify the central issue and deal with that issue while filling in minor information gaps with reasonable assumptions.

The first case or two you write may perhaps take you more time than you believe the process is worth. You may find, however, that writing cases is much like *doing* cases—and in fact much like making decisions—in that your performance improves with practice. The more you do, the better you become at doing it.

Index

A

Acquisition of supplies, 110-111
Alternatives to *Casebook,* 6
Anger, 33, 102-103
Apprehension, 34
Attendance problem, 58
Attitudes, employee, 72-73, 95-96,
  101-103, 106-107, 111-112, 117
Authority, resistance to, 39, 93

B

Blame, 73, 77

C

Casebook
  alphabetical listing of cases in,
    27-30
  classification of cases in, 25-30
  emphases in, 11-12, 76
  forced-choice pair analysis, use of
    in, 14-18
  topic numbering and cross-reference
    in, 26-27
  topics, choice of, 12-13
  topic survey for, 13-15, 18-21
  uses of, 1-3
Cases
  appropriateness of, analysis of, 32

fictional, 190-191
  relevance of, to current problems,
    31
  simplicity of, 191
  sources of material for, 189-190
Case study method, 185-188
Change, definition of, 13
Characteristics, desirable human, 7
Classroom situation, group oriented
  activities and, 1
Coffee break, abuse of, 85-86
Common sense in decision making,
  92-93
Communication, 58-59, 67, 69,
  109-110, 129
  and change in management, 59-60,
    98-99, 111-113
  confidentiality and, 50-51, 82, 108,
    115-118
  and delegation of responsibility,
    60-61, 62-64, 105-107, 127-128
  with difficult superior, 39-40, 45-47,
    70
  and disciplinary problems, 58,
    85-88, 96-97, 117, 134-135
  distortion of, 40-41, 48-50
  failure of, 52-56, 62-64
  hours assigned and, 80-85
  interdepartmental, 39-40, 42-43,
    110-111
  and leadership, 43-47

management functions and, 43-45,
    47-48, 57, 91-93, 97-98, 122-126
morale and, 41-42, 72-77, 88-90
and motivation, 43-45
organizational problems and,
    98-107, 118-120, 130-131, 133-134
as people problem, 23, 79
promotions and, 37-38, 40-41,
    103-104, 114-115
written, 118, 149-164
Compassion, 7, 9
Conditions for hiring, 130
Confidentiality of information, 50-51,
    82, 108, 115-118
Conscience, 79
Continuing education, 3
Controlling, as management skill,
    123, 125-126
Co-ordinating, as management skill,
    123, 125-126
Cost control, 78-79
Courage, 7-8
Creativity, 13
Criticism and discipline, 53-57, 73,
    94-95
    for inappropriate behavior, 72-73,
        95-96, 101-103, 117
    for poor performance, 52-53, 57-59,
        73, 93

D

Decision making
    and disciplinary action, 90-92,
        96-97
    in-basket exercise and, 152
    limitations on, 70-72, 75-76, 93,
        115-118
    priorities and, 132
    and union contract breach, 68-69
Delegation of responsibility
    and appointing supervisors, 103-104
    conditions for, 129-130
    in-basket exercise and, 152-157
    mistakes in, 42-43, 52-53, 59-64,

97-98, 105-106, 127-128
    for non-managerial duties, 106-107
    re-assignment by a higher authority
        and, 64-65
    to volunteers, 61-62
Dependability, as management skill,
    123, 125-126
Disappointment, 33
Disciplinary action, 8, 93, 95-96
Distortion of communication, 40-41,
    48-50

E

Educational programs, 4, 11
Efficiency, 99
Employee
    discipline, 95-96
    motivation, 13
Equipment, acquisition of, 110-111
Expectations, frustrated, 114-115
Expenses, 79

F

Fairness, 112-113
Films, problems with use of, 4
Firing, 53-56

G

General management practice
    basic management functions and,
        122-126, 129-130
    systems problems and, 42-43
Grapevine, 40-41
Group activities, 4

H

Hiring, 53-56, 66-68
    under false pretenses, 67
    from outside, employee resentment

against, 38
probation period and, 94-95
roles of supervisors and personnel
department in, 116-117
use of forbidden information in, 60
Hours, 80-85
Human relations movement, 10

I

Information, 66, 82
In-basket exercise, 149-164
Individual consideration, supervisory
problems and, 5
Inservice education, 71
Institutional change, 98-99
Insubordination, 96
Interdepartmental communication,
39-40, 42-43, 110-111
Interpersonal relations, 137-147
and motivation, 50-51
open-ended case involving, 144

L

Labor relations, 56-57, 68-69, 138
Leadership, 8, 129-130
basic management functions and,
122-123
change and, 98-99, 111-112
communication and, 43-47
confidentiality and, 82, 108,
129-130
delegation of responsibility and,
60-61, 105-106
employee attitude and, 37-41,
58-59, 82-84
organization and, 118-120, 132
style of, 23, 70, 129
unions and, 69
Line function, 117

M

Maintenance, plant, 98-99
Management, 5, 12, 24, 65, 112-114
and communication, 43-45, 47-48,
52, 91-93, 97-98, 122-126
and delegation, 97-98
functions and leadership, 122-123
practice, 99
problems, 102
Management, change in, 110-111
and communication, 59-60, 98-99,
111-113, 118
employee attitude and, 40-41,
112-114
incompetent advisor and, 70-72
organization and, 39, 113-114,
118-127, 130-131
priorities of new supervisor and,
132
as result of high turnover, 37
termination of employment and,
90-92
unexpected, 111-112
Medical records, handling of, 62-64
Meetings
confrontational situations in, 41-42
group criticism and, 57
group unwillingness to participate
in, 41-42
multiple departmental involvement
in, 39-40
punctuality and, 117
Methods, improvement of, 114-115
cost cutting and, 78-79
definition of, 13
office practice and, 121-123
organizational bottlenecks and,
118-120
for pre-admission scheduling, 118
pressure and, 115-116
resistance to, 112-113
Morale, 40-42, 72-77, 88-90, 99
Motivation, employee
change and, 111-113

communication and, 40-42, 48-50, 72-77, 88-90
employee attitude and, 37-38, 40-42, 72-73, 114-115
equipment acquisition and, 110-111
insufficient preparation and, 127-128
interpersonal relations and, 50-51
productivity and, 117
supervisor's role in, 24, 43-45, 73, 106-107
unrewarded, 62-64
volunteers and, 61-62

N

Negligence, discipline for act of, 58-59

O

Office practice, 121-127
One-to-one communication, definition of, 13
Operational procedure, 130-131
Organizational bottleneck, 98-101, 118-120
Organizational weaknesses, 102-103
Organizing, as management skill, 123, 125-126
Outside hiring, employee resentment against, 37-39, 41
Overtime, 56-57, 68-69

P

People problems, 66, 79-80, 87-88
attendance and, 58
coffee break abuse and, 85-86
communication and, 23, 48-50, 79
confidentiality and, 50-51, 82, 103

employee attitude and, 72-73, 88-90, 107, 114-115
hours and, 80-81, 84-85
organization and, 90-92, 98-103
personal characteristics and, 52-53, 58-59, 70-73, 75-78, 117
pressure and, 115-116
supervisor's job and, 43-45, 47-48, 79, 105-107, 123-126
with volunteers, 61-62
warnings and, 96-97
Personal business on company time, 87-88
Personal days, abuses of, 58
Personal effectiveness
communication and, 45-47
drop-in visitor problem and, 134-135
hiring conditions and, 129-130
insufficient preparation and, 127-128
organization and, 99-103, 121-127, 130-131
priorities and, 132-134
supervisor's job and, 97, 103-107, 122-126, 129
value of time and, 109-110
Personal supervisory effectiveness, definition of, 13
Personnel function, 117, 138
Planning, 123, 125-126, 152-157
Pre-admission procedure, 118
Preparation, insufficient, 127-128
Presentations, variety of, 3-4
Pressure, 115-116
Principles of management, 3, 5
Probation period, 94-95
Problem-solving, 185-187
Productivity, 120-121
Priorities, communication of, 132-134
Promotion
communication and, 37-38, 40-41, 103-104, 114-115
within structure of organization, 38
"Pulling away", 129, 166-168
Punctuality, 117

Q

Questions
concerning relations with
employees, 169-176, 179
higher management, 176-183
others, 178
example of, 166-168
uses of, 165-166

R

Rejection, 34
Relief, 33
Relocation, job, 112-113
Replacement, 111-112
Reports, 127-128
Resentment, 39
Respect, 109-110
Responsibility, motivation and, 73
Role-plays, in classroom situation, 1
Rules and policies, 66, 87-88
and abuse of coffee break, 85-86
employee attitudes and, 88-90,
95-96
for hiring, 116-117
hours and, 80-85, 95-96, 116-117
lenient application of, 53-56
unions and, 68-69
Rumors, 48-50

S

Scheduling, 58, 60-61, 130-131
Shift, choice of, 82-84
Sick time, 58
Small-group management
development activity, *Casebook*
and, 3
Solutions, provided by case study
method, 5
Staff functions, 117

Subordinate supervisors, appointment
of, 103-104
Supervisor, 6-10
communication and, 39-40, 45-47,
70
leadership and, 23
motivation and, 8, 24
weakness in, 10
Supervisory authority, 87-88
confidentiality and, 108
employee attitude and, 39-40, 70,
85-86, 88-90, 95-96, 109-110
in hiring, 116-117
institutional change and, 98-99
interpersonal relations and, 50-51
limits to, 92-93
organization and, 42-43, 59-60,
82-84, 94-95, 99-101
personal relationships versus, 79
supervisor's job and, 45-47, 64-65,
76-77, 97-98, 103-104
termination of employment and,
90-92
truth versus, 47-48
unions and, 68-69
warnings and, 96-97
work hours and, 80-81
Supervisory development, 3, 150
Supervisory problems, 22
Supervisory skills, 11
Supervisory topic-preference survey,
18-20
Supervisory training, 1-6

T

Tardiness, 53-56
Termination of employment, 90-92
Textbook approach, traditional,
contrasted with *Casebook*, 5-6
Time, 132-134
Time management, 109-110, 130-135
Transfers, job, 59-60

U

Unions, 13, 68-69

V

Villain, need to be liked and
  role of, 8
Visitors, drop-in, 134-135
Visual aids, use of, 4

Volunteers, use of, 62

W

Wage structure, inequities in, 37-38
Warnings for unsatisfactory
  performance, 96-97
Work hats, 80
Work methods, 114
Written communication, 13, 118,
  149-167